WHOLE BODY RESET DIET COOKBOOK

1200-Day Delicious Recipes and a 28-Day Meal Plan to Lose Weight, Get the Flat Belly, and Live Healthier in Your Midlife and Beyond

Theresa Martinez

Table Of Content

4

INTRODUCTION

In 2012, Harley Pasternak, a celebrity fitness trainer who co-hosted ABC's daytime talk show "The Revolution," developed the Body Reset Diet. Pasternak has worked with many A-listers, including Ariana Grande, Alicia Keys, Lady Gaga, Gwyneth Paltrow, Adam Levine, Megan Fox, Rihanna, Kanye West, Bono, and Katy Perry.

The diet is divided into three phases, each lasting five days, and the first phase consists mostly of drinking smoothies before reintroducing solid foods. First, you'll only be consuming smoothies for your meals. That means you'll only be having smoothies as part of your meals throughout the first phase. Milk or Greek yoghurt is a wonderful source of protein, and white smoothies are a fantastic way to get it. For a quick rush of energy, try a red smoothie made with fruits, while a green smoothie made with veggies will keep you satisfied until dinnertime. A salad, sandwich or stir-fry can be substituted for one of your two smoothies each day during the second phase of the diet. Finally, in phase three, a substantial meal is substituted for one of the two smoothies.

It's a 15-day experiment to see if a low-calorie plant-based diet consisting mostly of smoothies may educate your body to burn calories more effectively while you sleep. With three days of resistance training a week, you'll be on your way to long-term weight loss.

There may be a greater food spending on the Body Reset Diet because you'll be eating many fruits and veggies. Since you won't be purchasing any meat or other solid foods for the first few weeks,

7

you may experience a drop in your shopping price. Instead of buying fresh produce, Pasternak says, you can buy most fruits and vegetables pre-frozen and save money on groceries.

On the Body Reset Diet, you're likely to shed a few pounds. Unfortunately, dietary data does not exist for this diet; however, consuming only smoothies made from fresh produce may provide a deficit in calories, which might lead to weight loss. Whether or whether you manage to lose the weight and keep it off is entirely up to you.

Vegetarianism and the Body Reset diet both adhere to similar principles. As a general rule, vegetarians tend to consume fewer calories and weigh less than their meat-eating counterparts and eat a greater number of fruits and vegetables. Fruit and vegetable-rich diets have been linked to greater health in the long term.

CHAPTER 1:

WHY WHOLE-BODY RESET DIET FOR A FLAT BELLY

Weight loss may be achieved by "eating more and exercising less" but losing weight with the Body Reset program. People who have tried and failed at other weight loss methods will benefit most from this one. Due to its low initial caloric intake, the Body Reset diet may rapidly reduce weight. A sensible workout routine is also emphasized in this guide. Even if you stick to a short-term diet, you won't get long-term results. One of the world's leading experts in nutritional science and fitness and author of The 5-Factor Diet, Harley Pasternak, devised a new diet called the Body Reset in 2013. The diet's foundation is straightforward: Smoothies are a great way to jumpstart a weight reduction program. You can gradually transition to a better diet that still incorporates smoothies (just fewer of them). The Body Reset program also includes a workout regimen. The Body Reset plan claims to kick-start your metabolism and help you lose weight by having you consume smoothies primarily for 15 days. Even if you lose a little weight while on a diet, most experts believe you'll gain it back once the program is over. The strategy is short-term and lacks long-term direction. It is unsustainable.

The Body Reset program consists of three five-day phases: Phase I, where you only drink smoothies and snacks; Phase II, where you only consume smoothies and one meal and two snacks per day; and Phase III, when you only consume one smoothie per day and two meals and two snacks per day.

There will be two "free" meals a week during the "maintenance" phase when you can eat and drink as much as you like after the third five-day phase. Nuts, seeds, and avocados are included in the diet, prioritising low-fat foods. "Pretty much any fruit or vegetable you can name" are the words the company uses to describe its smoothies, made with milk protein and high-fibre carbs.

The Body Reset system's most significant component is smoothies. It's white for breakfast, red for lunch, and green for dinner (dinner). An apple, a pear, or a nectarine are all staples in the basic white smoothie. Bananas and almonds are also common ingredients. One scoop of protein powder, one tablespoon of ground flaxseed, and half an orange are needed to make one of these smoothies. Fruits and vegetables such as spinach, kale, romaine lettuce, pear, and grapes, together with yoghurt, avocado, and lime juice, make up a green smoothie. Each type of smoothie has its own set of six recipes. But if you'd rather create your own, there are also suggestions for replacements (such as almonds in avocado or tofu in place of Greek yoghurt). Snacks on the Body Reset diet should consist of high-fibre fruits and vegetables. When it comes to fruits like apples and pears, it's also crucial to consume their skins rather than peel them.

Pasternak stresses the need for frequent little meals to maintain a steady blood sugar level and prevent overeating when it comes to eating. The first two phases of the diet are likely to cause you to feel hungry.

Also, the diet encourages choosing healthy food choices. For example, you need to have a plan in place to avoid snacking on junk food when you're hungry and make the most of your calorie intake. Pasternak suggests "S-meals" in phases II and III of the regimen. Scrambles, scramble-like dishes such as eggs and bacon are included in the S category.

In addition to the diet, there is a simple workout regimen included. To begin, aim to walk at least 10,000 steps every day. The walking is supplemented with strength training three days per week during the second phase. Five days a week of weight exercise and at least 10,000 daily steps are required in the third phase. The Body Reset diet requires a high-quality blender to succeed. To acquire the same volume of food, juicing necessitates more productive. Still, blending uses all of the fibrous components of the fruits and vegetables, which contain most nutrients, making them simpler to consume.

CHAPTER 2:

THE WHOLE BODY RESET WEIGHT LOSS PROGRAM

It's hard to begin a diet because of the terrible goodbyes we may have to say goodbye to our favourite meals or the uncertainty about whether we'll be able to maintain our new waistline. Yet, according to a March 2017 research published in the Journal of the American Medical Association, fewer Americans than ever are attempting to lose weight. This might be one of the reasons. A 15-day, low-exercise detox called the Body Reset diet promises to help people lose weight and keep it off if they stick to it for 15 days.

Body Reset, a smoothie-based diet, was developed by celebrity trainer and author Harley Pasternak in 2013 to simplify diets. The liquid diet, popularized by celebrities like Kim Kardashian and Rhianna, is based on the idea that wonderful cuisine may be enjoyed in moderation while promoting regular physical activity and water consumption. Despite appearing to leave the body with nothing, the liquid meals include the right quantities of all the dietary categories (except solid food, of course).

As tempting as it may be to sip smoothies every day, there are several important considerations to keep in mind before pulling out your blender. The Body Reset program is broken into three five-day periods, like the South Beach Diet or the Whole30. Although the meals in each phase change, smoothies remain the primary source of nutrition. Pasternak argues that the primary benefit of a smoothie-based diet is its ease of use. It's usually a container for a variety of different substances. The smoothies all have "identical calorie value," "fibre, protein, and good fats."

Carbs, protein, and fibre are Pasternak's "Holy Trinity of metabolism," and this idea is the focus of the Body Reset diet (and the hoopla around it). When these nutrients are combined with smaller amounts throughout the day and a goal step count is attained, Body Reset claims to reset metabolism in a way that helps maintain weight reduction after the program is complete.

There are two allowed "crunchy snacks" every day that are high in fibre, protein, and healthy fats and the daily smoothies. As you progress through the diet, you'll gradually begin to eat solid foods known as "S" (single-dish) meals (scramble, salad, stir fry, sandwich, or soup). Avoid overeating by sticking to a single-item meal. For the "Holy Trinity" and the consumption of lesser quantities, that's all you need.

Exercise is the final way to increase your metabolism. Not in the gym, I'll tell you that right now. Pasternak recommends that you walk 10,000 steps every day, no matter what time of day or how you do it. According to the American Heart Association, this is also the suggested step count for those who want to lower their risk of heart disease. Aside from these two five-minute resistance workouts, Pasternak also recommends three times a week to do modified push-ups or triceps dips.

There are three smoothies for breakfast, lunch, and supper for the first five days. Color-coded to represent the five primary food groups recommended by the United States Department of Agriculture, these smoothies are grouped into three distinct categories (USDA). Yoghurt and whole milk are two protein-rich ingredients found in the white morning smoothie. Various fruits are included in this vibrant crimson lunchtime smoothie. For supper, the green smoothie has all the veggies you need for a healthy diet. As a bonus, you'll have two "crunchy snacks" full of protein and fibre to munch on between your three smoothies, which you'll need to make ahead of time. For the second five days of the solid-food detox, your primary source of nutrition will be smoothies, as was the case in the first phase. In the second phase, smoothies are replaced with "S" meals to reintroduce solid foods to your diet. It doesn't matter if you have an "S" dinner or a smoothie. However, Pasternak advises you to proceed with prudence. "You may use your usual meals to enhance it," he says. Just include some green veggies if you don't have time to create a green smoothie for supper.

However, how probable will your metabolism be improved sufficiently to continue controlling continuous weight reduction after the diet? Kennedy's response: "Not probable at all, to be honest."

In certain cases, she says, "It may also mean 15 days when you came off, and you did pretty well, and then you return to eating the way you've always eaten." While Pasternak relies on dieters to continue eating following the Body Reset diet after the program is finished, That is, by following the suggested step counts, grazing patterns, nutritionally-balanced food groupings, and single-item meals. "Your life," he explains, "is the third phase." However, Kennedy thinks that things are more complicated than that. Even though Body Reset's quick weight reduction may be achieved, a person's resolve to maintain such extensive lifestyle modifications (such as walking to the most remote supermarket for 10,000 steps) will not likely hold. Instead, Kennedy recommends adopting smaller, more manageable lifestyle adjustments to lose weight, such as increasing your veggies and lean protein intake and reducing your portion sizes.

According to the National Center for Complementary and Integrative Health, a "detox" or "cleanse" is characterized by removing solid food from the body, which is not regarded as a deficiency of nutrients. (4) Dietitians like Kennedy generally advise against following such rigid dietary regimens. Kennedy asserts that the body "never needs a cleanse." In other words, we don't need to interfere with the body's natural detoxification processes. The liver, kidneys, and lungs' job is to eliminate toxins from the body when they are in good working order.

Pasternak maintains that the Body Reset diet is not a "cleanse," even though it may offer all five USDA food categories. You'll be OK as long as you're paying attention to what you're putting in your smoothies. There are numerous smoothies made by Pasternak that feature at least one piece of fruit, which might add up to seven servings of fruit each day. According to Kennedy, "that's more than double the typical recommended" and "makes it an extremely horrible fit for someone with diabetes."

CHAPTER 3:

BENEFITS OF THE WHOLE BODY RESET PROGRAM

Losing weight can be a difficult process that needs a lot of effort, perseverance, and commitment. The best method to lose weight is to change your food, lifestyle, and exercise habits rather than relying on fad diets and fat-burning products. If you want to lose weight and improve your general health, you may take several basic actions.

Exercises that focus on strengthening your muscles are known as strength training. Over time, it improves muscle growth and strength, and lifting weights is a common method.

According to studies, strength training provides several health advantages, especially when it comes to fat loss. Resistance exercise for at least four weeks has been shown to help reduce body fat by an average of 1.46 per cent, according to an analysis of 58 research. As a result, it may help you lose weight and visceral fat, which is fat that encircles your inside organs. Another study found that teenagers with obesity who did 5 months of strength training were more likely to lose weight than those who did aerobic exercise alone. As a result, resistance exercise may help you burn more calories at rest by preserving fat-free muscle. Resistance training increased people's resting metabolic rate compared to a control group, but the aerobic exercise had no impact. Strength training may be begun by doing bodyweight exercises, lifting weights, and utilizing gym equipment.

Reduce your appetite and enhance fat burning by increasing your intake of protein-rich meals. Studies have linked a higher intake of high-quality protein to a decreased risk of obesity and excess body fat. In addition, according to other studies, high protein diets have been shown to assist in maintaining muscle mass and metabolism during weight reduction. Increasing your protein consumption may also help you feel fuller, reduce appetite, and consume fewer calories, contributing to a healthy weight reduction strategy. A few portions of high-protein meals will help you get the protein you need each day. Tofu, beans, and dairy products like milk and cheese are all examples of protein-rich foods.

An easy method to help you lose weight and keep it off is to go to bed earlier or set your alarm clock a little later. Weight reduction is linked to a healthy amount of sleep, according to several research. For example, 10-year research found that young women who slept less than six hours a night were more likely to become obese. Another small research found that dieters on a low-calorie diet lost less fat when they slept one hour less each night than those in the control group. Other studies have shown that sleep deprivation may change hunger hormones, resulting in an increased appetite and an increased risk of obesity.

Most studies link at least seven hours of sleep a night to the best positive outcomes for weight loss and overall health. Stick to a regular sleep schedule, restrict your evening coffee intake, and avoid using electronic devices an hour or two before you go to bed if you want to promote a healthy sleep cycle. Healthy fats can help you avoid weight gain, even if it seems paradoxical. People who ate more olive oil and almonds as part of a Mediterranean diet lost more weight in the long run than those who ate less fat.

Another study found that diets fortified with olive oil resulted in better weight loss and fat belly reductions than diets that did not include olive oil. Trans fats, a kind of lipid commonly found in fried and processed foods, have been linked to an elevated risk of long-term obesity. Nutritious fats like olive oil, coconut oil, avocados, almonds, and seeds are a few examples. Maintain a healthy fat intake, but remember that it's still heavy in calories. Opt for the healthier alternatives above instead of the fried and processed fare, processed ingredients, and refined oils that you'd normally consume more of. One of the simplest methods to encourage long-term, sustained fat reduction is to swap out sugary drinks for healthy alternatives.

Sugar-sweetened drinks like soda, for example, are frequently high in calories and low in nutrients. You may be more likely to overeat if you drink alcohol since it has a lot of calories and can weaken your inhibitions. Sugar-sweetened drinks and alcohol have been linked to an increased risk of obesity. Instead, drink water or green tea, which are both calorie-free. After this little trial, 14 young men were more satisfied and less hungry when they drank 1 pint (570 mL) of water before eating. Caffeine and antioxidants in green tea, on the other hand, have the potential to improve fat burning and metabolism.

CHAPTER 4:

THE PRINCIPLES OF THE WHOLE BODY RESET PROGRAM

Calories measure the quantity of energy in a meal or beverage. Fat is stored in our bodies when we eat or drink more calories than we expend. If this trend continues, we run the risk of gaining excess weight. An average man's daily caloric requirement to maintain a healthy weight is around 2,500 kcal (10,500 kJ). Daily caloric intake for an average female is around 2,000kcal (8,400kJ). Different factors such as the individual's size and amount of physical activity influence these numbers. Our bodies require energy to keep us alive and our organs operating properly. Consuming food and beverages provide our bodies with energy. However, everyday activities such as breathing and jogging deplete our bodies with this energy.

There must be a balance between what we eat and how much exercise we do to keep a steady weight. Maintaining a good energy balance is a key component of a nutritious diet.

We utilize more energy when we engage in more physical exercise. Don't worry if you use a lot of energy every day. Simply reduce your daily caloric intake from here on out. The calorie content of food and drink might assist you in avoiding overeating. Calorie information may be found on the packaging of many store-bought items. In the "Energy" section, you'll find this information. Kcals and kJ are commonly used to describe the calorie content of food, which may be expressed as either kilocalories or kilojoules.

If you want to write 1,000 calories as 1,000kcals, you'll need the word kilocalorie. The metric unit of measure for calories is kilojoules. Calories are multiplied by 4.2 to get kilojoules of energy. The calorie content of a meal or drink may be compared by looking at the label, which will tell you how many calories are in 100 grams or 100 millilitres.

It's common practice to provide the number of calories in a serving on food labels. However, remember that the manufacturer's definition of a portion may differ from yours, so the piece you serve yourself may be higher in calories. Calorie counts might help you figure out how much a certain item contributes to your daily caloric needs.

Calorie counters for PCs and mobile phones may be found in various places online and on the internet. Many of these are available for free download and use. The NHS recommends keeping a food diary to keep track of your daily caloric intake. If you're dining out and want to keep an eye on your caloric intake, you can look it up on the menu at some establishments. Per serving or per meal, calories should be counted.

Size and age affect how many calories people burn when engaging in a particular physical activity. You'll burn more calories if you exercise aggressively. Fast walking, for example, burns more calories than slow walking. To gain weight, you may eat and drink more calories than your body needs. The only way to lose weight is to burn more calories than you ingest continuously.

CHAPTER 5:

THE MAGIC OF PROTEIN TIMING IN NUTRITION

Many years of scientific investigation into diet and weight loss have yielded a few critical findings on what it takes to win the war against obesity. A person's good eating habits are more essential than the amount of time they spend at the gym when shedding pounds. First of all, there isn't just one diet that can help you get in shape, but rather a several different diets that will help you lose weight, keeping track of your calorie intake. One of the most important "levers" in a weight loss diet is the protein consumed. This book will help you sort through all of the conflicting information about protein and provide you with specific recommendations on how much to consume to achieve your weight loss goals. Protein is an essential macronutrient that plays a role in almost all body activities and functions. As an important ingredient for good health, it aids in muscle repair after exercise and aids in the maintenance of a healthy weight. An amino acid is a compound made up of carbon, hydrogen, oxygen, and nitrogen that is the basis for protein synthesis. A few of their many functions, proteins and amino acids help build and repair body tissues, manufacture enzymes and other cellular transporters, and more.

A daily protein intake of 1.6 to 2.2 grams per kilogram of body weight is recommended for weight loss (.73 and 1 grams per pound). If you want to lose weight, you should eat 2.2-3.4 grams of protein per kilogram (1-1.5 grams per pound). BMI above 30 or a body fat percentage exceeding 25-30 per cent is my realistic guideline for folks. It makes more sense to tailor your protein intake to your desired weight loss. Additionally, protein aids in weight reduction by preserving lean body mass during periods of calorie restriction, which is another advantage.

Low protein consumption (1.0 grams per kilogram per day) and high protein intake (2.3 grams per kilogram per day) were examined in a short-term calorie deficit research to see how they affected lean body mass. Muscle mass loss in the low protein group was 1.6 kilograms (3.5 pounds), whereas muscle mass loss in the high protein group averaged 0.3 kilograms (0.6 pounds). It was also discovered in another comparable study that the two higher intakes (2.4 and 1.6 g/kg per day) preserved greater lean body mass than the 0.8 g/kg per day diet. However, they also observed that 2.4 g/kg/day was no better than 1.6 g/kg/day.

A daily protein consumption of 1.6 grams per kilogram of body weight, or.73 grams of protein per pound, is now the recommended daily objective for protein intake during times of weight reduction to preserve lean body mass. More energy is eaten than is exerted when trying to lose weight. As a result, it's critical to keep the number of extra calories stored as fat to a minimum. The three macronutrients (proteins, carbs, and fats) are processed differently by the body. The metabolic process that protein goes through to be stored as fat is somewhat distinct from the processes that carbs and other forms of protein go through.

CHAPTER 6:

THE BENEFITS OF THE WHOLE BODY RESET DIET

Keeping a trim midsection does more than just improve your appearance; it may also extend your life. Heart disease, diabetes, and possibly cancer are all associated with having a larger waistline. Being overweight or obese can negatively affect blood vessel function and sleep quality. When dieting, you can't precisely target abdominal fat. You can't see visceral fat, a form of fat in your abdomen that increases your risk of heart disease and stroke, but decreasing weight overall can help lower your waistline and lessen this harmful layer of visceral fat. If you're trying to lose weight and keep it off for six months, you'll lose 10 more pounds on a low-carbohydrate diet over a low-fat diet—28.9 pounds to 18.7 pounds, according to Johns Hopkins researchers. Stewart claims that the low-carb diet also contributed to better-quality weight reduction. Losing weight might reduce fat, but it can also lead to muscle loss, which is undesirable. Both diets resulted in a fat loss of 2 to 3 pounds, but the low-carbohydrate diet resulted in a higher fat loss percentage.

The most important thing, according to Stewart, is to choose a diet that you can adhere to. Low-carbohydrate diets don't require calorie tracking because they make better meal choices. Diets low in carbohydrates and rich in fibre, such as whole grains, legumes, poultry, fish, and meat, tend to emphasize lower-carbohydrate and higher-protein alternatives.

Abdominal fat can be lost by regular exercise. "exercise is one of the best investments you can make " in terms of body composition," adds Stewart. There's a lot of evidence that exercise helps you lose weight because it lowers insulin levels and enables your liver to burn up the fat stored in your abdominal area, where most of your visceral fat is located. How much exercise you need for weight reduction depends on your goals. Moderate-to-vigorous exercise for 30 to 60 minutes five days a week is a reasonable goal for most people. At rest and when exercising, you burn more calories when you add moderate strength training to your aerobic exercise regimen. Brands can be compared and contrasted. Stewart points out that while some yoghurts advertise that they are reduced in fat, they are heavier in carbohydrates and added sugars. High-fat and high-calorie foods like gravy and salad dressings are typically found in these dishes.

The trans fats added to sugar and salt or sodium found in packaged products and snack meals make it harder to lose weight.

Instead of obsessing over your weight, pay attention to how your clothes fit. The number on the bathroom scale may not move much, but your jeans will be tighter as you gain muscle and shed fat. That's a more telling sign of development than anything else I could think of. If you're a woman, your waistline should be no more than 35 inches, and if you're a male, it should be no more than 40 inches. Research suggests that if your friends and family are doing the same, you're more likely to eat healthily and exercise more frequently. A hormone produced in your pancreas by cells. As a result of eating, insulin assists your body in storing the glucose (sugar) it produces. As a person with diabetes, your pancreas may not produce enough insulin; therefore, you may be prescribed medication to assist your liver produce more or increasing insulin sensitivity in your muscles, depending on your condition. As a last resort, you may be given insulin injections.

Blood travels through the body through a network of arteries, capillaries, and veins. Small, thin-walled capillaries transport oxygen and nutrients to cells and remove waste products, including carbon dioxide, from the bloodstream. Carbon dioxide is exhaled as you exhale through your lungs and heart, which get the blood from the capillaries. The veins in your body transport oxygen-rich blood away from your heart. Arteries resemble long, thin tubes. They consist of three layers: a tough, muscle-filled middle layer and a smooth inner wall that makes blood flow easier. Muscles contract and extend to facilitate blood flow. According to a 2012 study by Johns Hopkins researchers, a diet low in fat and carbs can enhance arterial health. Those on the low-carb diet lost more weight and did so more quickly after six months. The arteries improved as the weight dropped, especially when the belly fat shrunk. This allowed more blood to flow through the arteries. According to a new study, there is no need to eliminate all fat from your diet to reduce abdominal fat. Having a healthy heart appears to be a simple matter of decreasing weight and exercising.

CHAPTER 7:

WHAT TO EXPECT FROM THE WHOLE BODY RESET DIET

People who consume a protein-rich diet have a better chance of losing weight because they are less likely to overeat. In addition, when paired with regular exercise, a high-protein diet can aid in developing lean muscle. Lean muscle aids in weight loss by increasing the rate at which calories are burned throughout the day. This is a list of some of the greatest high-protein meals for weight loss you can eat. A high-protein diet is effective in helping people lose weight.

There is a reduction in hunger hormones and cravings, increased fullness, and increased calories expended, among other things. However, choosing the optimal protein for weight reduction might be tough when so many alternatives for increasing protein consumption. This book discusses the various forms of protein and their impact on weight reduction. Even without limiting calories or other nutrients, high-protein diets have resulted in weight loss. Over 12 weeks, overweight persons who raised their protein consumption from 15% to 30% of their daily calories shed 11 pounds (5 kg).

It has also been found that high-protein diets positively impact weight loss and lean muscle mass. Maintaining your weight reduction may be easier if you eat a lot of protein. According to one study, those who ate 18 per cent more protein per day than they did 15 per cent of the time saw a 50 per cent reduced rate of weight gain. It's been shown that consuming foods high in protein frequently will help you lose weight.

An egg-based diet has been shown to minimize total daily caloric consumption by making you feel satiated for longer. It has also been shown that eating protein-rich nuts, beans, and legumes regularly will help you maintain or even shed pounds. Furthermore, both animal- and plant-based protein sources appear to be equally effective in promoting weight reduction. According to research, overweight people lost the same amount of weight on either a plant-protein-heavy diet or an animal-protein-heavy diet. Similar findings were made in other research. There were weight reduction, hunger management, and food intake advantages to high plant-based protein diets compared to high animal-based protein diets.

CHAPTER 8:

THE THREE PHASES OF THE WHOLE BODY RESET DIET

Harley Pasternak is a well-known personal trainer with a deep understanding of nutrition and health. When he came up with the body reset diet and the notion of just depending on smoothies and short meals, he was the one who came up with it. Many individuals in this country have been trying to lose weight for a long time and haven't been seeing much progress or inspiration; therefore, Harley Pasternak believes that the more results you see regularly, the more likely you are to stick to a diet in the long run (received scientific support)

There are three phases to the 15-day regimen. To jumpstart weight reduction in the first five days, the body reset diet uses meal plans with extremely low caloric intake, such as 1200 to 1400 calories. A basic exercise regimen, such as walking 10,000 steps or doing light exercise at home, will be recommended to you to complement your eating plan.

During Phase 1 (for the first 5 days), your body undergoes a slew of tough changes to maintain. You're expected to drink smoothies for breakfast, lunch, and supper. Two low-calorie snacks each day are permitted. To be considered physically active, you need to walk 10,000 steps a day.

Phase 2 (the next 5 days): You will have to substitute any two meals with a smoothie, which means that you can consume one solid-state dinner and two snacks. As for physical activity, you must walk 10,000 steps a day and perform five minutes of weight training using various exercises.

During Phase 3 (Last 5 Days), you will only be consuming one smoothie per day, and you will also be eating two low-calorie meals and two snacks each day. On the third day, you'll walk 10,000 steps and do 5 minutes of weight training, alternating between 4 different exercises each time. After following this diet plan, you will notice a noticeable improvement in your physique. After 15 days, you may be wondering what to do next. A lot of folks make the same error. Most individuals will only follow a diet for 15 days before returning to their old eating habits, putting their bodies and digestive systems under great strain.

As soon as you've completed the usual 15-day body reset diet, you must return to your 3-phase diet. The only thing you're allowed to do is provide complimentary meals twice each week. As a reward for your perseverance and hard work, you can eat whatever you want twice a week. Because you won't feel deprived anymore, you won't be tempted to binge eat, which happens when you place undue pressure on your body and deny it the things it craves. You can continue to follow the third phase of the body reset diet for the rest of your life once the 15-day period has ended.

CHAPTER 9: DRINKS & SMOOTHIES

Virgin Mary Smoothies

Preparation Time: 10 minutes
Cooking Time: 15 minutes
Servings: 1

Ingredients:
- 1 can of whole peeled tomatoes
- One stalk of celery, sliced
- One medium carrot, sliced
- One teaspoon of Worcestershire sauce
- One teaspoon of prepared horseradish, or more to taste
- ¼ teaspoon hot sauce
- 1 cup ice cubes

Directions:
- ➢ Combine the tomatoes, celery, carrots, Worcestershire sauce, horseradish, and spicy sauce in a blender until the mixture is completely smooth. Add ice cubes and mix until completely frothy.

Secret Ingredient Smoothie

Preparation Time: 10 minutes
Cooking Time: 15 minutes
Servings: 1

Ingredients:
- 3 cups chopped romaine lettuce
- ⅓ cup milk, or more as needed
- Four frozen strawberries or more to taste
- One frozen banana, cut into chunks
- ¼ teaspoon vanilla extract, or to taste (Optional)

Directions:
- ➢ Blend romaine lettuce with enough milk to thoroughly cover it in a blender pitcher; turn on High and blend until smooth.
- ➢ To avoid over-blending, add one strawberry at a time to the blender while it is still running on High. You may do the same thing with the bananas as with strawberries. Add more milk to thin the smoothie and ensure that it blends correctly. Add a splash of vanilla extract to taste.

Crunchy Pineapple Smoothie

Preparation Time: 10 minutes
Cooking Time: 15 minutes
Servings: 1

Ingredients:
- 1 cup boiling water
- 1 (2 g) bag green tea bag
- One large orange, peeled
- 1 cup pineapple chunks
- One kiwi fruit, peeled
- Three tablespoons of non-fat Greek yoghurt

Directions:
- ➢ In a bowl, combine boiling water and green tea; steep for 5 minutes.
- ➢ In a blender, combine the orange, pineapple, and kiwi fruit. Remove the tea bag from the tea and add the tea to the orange mixture; blend. Blend in the yoghurt until smooth.

Blueberry and Spice Smoothie

Preparation Time: 10 minutes
Cooking Time: 15 minutes
Servings: 1

Ingredients:
- ¼ cup ice cubes, or as desired

- 1 cup low-fat vanilla yoghurt
- 1 cup of low-fat milk
- ½ cup frozen blueberries, or to taste
- One teaspoon of ground cinnamon
- One tablespoon white sugar, or to taste

Directions:
- ➢ Combine the rice, yoghurt, milk, blueberries, and cinnamon in a blender until crumbly. Blend until completely smooth. Blend after tasting the smoothie and adding the required quantity of sugar.

Vanilla Pumpkin Pie Smoothie

Preparation Time: 10 minutes
Cooking Time: 15 minutes
Servings: 1

Ingredients:
- 8 ounces pumpkin pie filling (such as Libby's®)
- 1 cup vanilla frozen yoghurt
- ½ cup ice
- ½ cup vanilla-flavoured soy milk
- One teaspoon of ground cinnamon
- One pinch of ground nutmeg
- ⅛ teaspoon vanilla extract

Directions:
- ➢ In a blender, combine pumpkin pie filling, frozen yoghurt, ice, soy milk, cinnamon, nutmeg, and vanilla extract; mix until smooth.

Avocado Smoothie

Preparation Time: 10 minutes
Cooking Time: 15 minutes
Servings: 1

Ingredients:
- One ripe avocado halved and pitted
- 1 cup milk
- ½ cup vanilla yoghurt
- Three tablespoons honey
- Eight ice cubes

Directions:
- ➢ In a blender, combine the avocado, milk, yoghurt, honey, and ice cubes; mix until smooth.

Ultimate Fruit Smoothie

Preparation Time: 10 minutes
Cooking Time: 15 minutes
Servings: 1

Ingredients:
- ½ cup 2% milk
- ½ cup orange juice
- ½ mango
- ½ fresh peach - peeled, pitted, and sliced
- ¼ cup fresh pineapple chunks
- Two strawberries

Directions:
- ➢ In a blender, combine milk, orange juice, mango, peach, pineapple, and strawberries until blended.

Avocado Smoothie

Preparation Time: 10 minutes
Cooking Time: 15 minutes
Servings: 1

Ingredients:

- 12 fluid ounces of unsweetened almond milk
- One avocado, peeled and pitted
- One tablespoon honey

Directions:

- In a blender, combine almond milk, avocado, and honey; mix until smooth.

Chocolate Peanut Butter Banana Smoothies

Preparation Time: 10 minutes
Cooking Time: 15 minutes
Servings: 1

Ingredients:

- 2 (3.25 ounce) cups Snack Pack® Chocolate Pudding
- Two tablespoons Peter Pan® Creamy Peanut Butter
- Two large ripe bananas, cut into pieces
- ¾ cup reduced-fat (2%) milk
- 1 cup ice cubes
- Reddi-wip® Chocolate Dairy Whipped Topping

Directions:

- Blend all ingredients, except the Reddi-Wip, in a blender container until smooth.
- Divide equally among four glasses and top with one serving Reddi-Wip. Serve right away.

Island Smoothie

Preparation Time: 10 minutes
Cooking Time: 15 minutes
Servings: 1

Ingredients:

- 1 cup ice
- 2 cups pineapple juice
- ½ cup ginger ale
- Three tablespoons of coconut milk
- One tablespoon of white sugar

Directions:

- In a blender, combine the ice, pineapple juice, ginger ale, coconut milk, and sugar; mix until smooth.

Acai Berry Smoothie

Preparation Time: 10 minutes
Cooking Time: 15 minutes
Servings: 1

Ingredients:

- 2 cups orange juice
- One banana, sliced
- ½ cup acai berry pulp
- 1 pinch white sugar, or to taste

Directions:

- Combine orange juice, banana, acai pulp, and sugar until smooth in a blender.

Strawberry Fields Smoothie

Preparation Time: 10 minutes
Cooking Time: 15 minutes
Servings: 1

Ingredients:

- 2 cups fresh spinach
- 2 cups frozen unsweetened strawberries
- 1 cup chopped cucumber
- Two carrots, chopped
- One banana, cut into chunks
- One apple, chopped
- ⅔ cup water
- ½ cup ice cubes, or as desired
- One tablespoon flax seed, or to taste (Optional)

Directions:

- In a blender, combine spinach, strawberries, cucumber, carrots, banana, apple, water, ice cubes, and flax seed until smooth.

Yam Smoothie

Preparation Time: 10 minutes
Cooking Time: 15 minutes
Servings: 1

Ingredients:

- Two medium yams
- 3 cups vanilla yoghurt
- 1 cup milk
- 2 cups ice cubes
- One teaspoon of white sugar
- One ripe banana, sliced

Directions:

- Place yams on a platter and prick with a fork. Microwave for 8 to 10 minutes, rotating once or until tender. Cool before peeling and dicing.
- Combine the yams, yoghurt, milk, ice cubes, sugar, and banana in a blender container. Blend until completely smooth.

Blue Grapefruit Smoothie

Preparation Time: 10 minutes
Cooking Time: 15 minutes
Servings: 1

Ingredients:

- One grapefruit - peeled, seeds removed, and white pith removed
- 1 cup rice milk
- 1 cup blueberries
- ½ cup vanilla yoghurt
- ½ cup rolled oats
- One banana
- One kiwi
- Three tablespoons of white sugar

Directions:

- In a blender, combine grapefruit, rice milk, blueberries, yoghurt, oats, banana, kiwi, and sugar until blended.

Quick Pina Colada Smoothie

Preparation Time: 10 minutes
Cooking Time: 15 minutes
Servings: 1

Ingredients:

- 1 cup pineapple juice
- ½ cup unsweetened coconut cream
- ¼ cup ice cubes, or as desired

Directions:

- Blend pineapple juice, coconut cream, and ice cubes in a high-powered blender for 30 to 40 seconds or until smooth.

Almond Butter Smoothie

Preparation Time: 10 minutes
Cooking Time: 15 minutes
Servings: 1

Ingredients:

- 1 ½ cups almond milk
- Two peeled bananas, frozen
- Four pitted dates
- Five tablespoons of almond butter
- One tablespoon of ground cinnamon
- One tablespoon of flax seeds
- ½ teaspoon ground nutmeg

Directions:

> In a blender, combine almond milk, bananas, dates, almond butter, cinnamon, flax seeds, and nutmeg until smooth.

Grapefruit Smoothie

Preparation Time: 10 minutes
Cooking Time: 15 minutes
Servings: 1

Ingredients:
- Three grapefruits, peeled and sectioned
- 1 cup cold water
- 3 ounces fresh spinach
- Six ice cubes
- 1 (1/2 inch) piece peeled fresh ginger
- One teaspoon of flax seeds

Directions:
> In a blender or NutriBullet®, combine grapefruit, water, spinach, ice cubes, ginger, and flax seeds until blended.

Summertime Fruit Smoothie

Preparation Time: 10 minutes
Cooking Time: 15 minutes
Servings: 1

Ingredients:
- 1 cup Greek yoghurt
- 1 ½ cups frozen sliced peaches
- 1 cup frozen raspberries
- 3 ½ tablespoons raspberry honey
- 3 cups ice
- 1 ½ cups pineapple chunks
- 1 cup watermelon chunks
- One banana

Directions:
> In a blender, combine yoghurt, peaches, raspberries, and honey until smooth; add ice, pineapple, watermelon, and banana. Blend until completely smooth.

Sour Smoothie

Preparation Time: 10 minutes
Cooking Time: 15 minutes
Servings: 1

Ingredients:
- 1 cup ice cubes
- One orange, peeled
- Two limes, peeled
- One lemon, peeled
- One kiwi peeled
- One teaspoon of honey or more to taste

Directions:
> Combine ice, orange, limes, lemon, kiwi, and honey in a blender until smooth.

Carrot-Banana Smoothie

Preparation Time: 10 minutes
Cooking Time: 15 minutes
Servings: 1

Ingredients:
- One banana
- 1 cup chopped cucumbers
- ⅔ cup chopped red bell pepper
- ½ cup ruby-red grapefruit juice
- ½ cup chopped carrots
- ice cubes

Directions:
> Fill a glass halfway with ice and pour the smoothie over it.

Strawberry Banana Breeze Smoothie

Preparation Time: 10 minutes
Cooking Time: 15 minutes
Servings: 1

Ingredients:
- One medium banana
- 1 ½ cup fresh strawberries
- 1 cup Almond Breeze Original or Unsweetened Original almond milk
- ½ cup fresh or juice packed pineapple
- One tablespoon of slivered or sliced almonds (optional)
- One teaspoon of flax seeds (Optional)

Directions:
> In a blender, combine all of the ingredients and puree until smooth.

Silky Strawberry Smoothie

Preparation Time: 10 minutes
Cooking Time: 15 minutes
Servings: 1

Ingredients:
- 1 cup fresh strawberries
- One banana, sliced
- 1 cup ice
- ½ cup silken tofu
- One teaspoon of agave nectar (optional)

Directions:
> Combine strawberries, banana, rice, tofu, and agave nectar in a blender until smooth.

Fruit Smoothie II

Preparation Time: 10 minutes
Cooking Time: 15 minutes
Servings: 1

Ingredients:
- 1 cup blueberries
- Two apples - peeled, cored and chopped
- 1 ½ cups raspberries
- ¾ cup seedless grapes
- Three tablespoons of white sugar
- One tray of ice cubes

Directions:
> Combine blueberries, apples, raspberries, grapes, sugar, and ice in a blender. Blend until completely smooth. Pour into serving glasses and serve.

Silky Strawberry Smoothie

Preparation Time: 10 minutes
Cooking Time: 15 minutes
Servings: 1

Ingredients:
- 1 cup fresh strawberries
- One banana, sliced
- 1 cup ice
- ½ cup silken tofu
- One teaspoon of agave nectar (optional)

Directions:
> Combine strawberries, banana, rice, tofu, and agave nectar in a blender until smooth.

Fruit Smoothie II

Preparation Time: 10 minutes
Cooking Time: 15 minutes
Servings: 1

Ingredients:
- ¾ cup raspberries, or to taste
- ½ cup plain fat-free Greek yoghurt

- ½ cup crushed ice
- One apricot - peeled, pitted, and chopped
- Two tablespoons honey
- One tablespoon of flax seeds
- One tablespoon of lemon juice

Directions:
- ➢ In a blender, combine raspberries, yoghurt, ice, apricot, honey, flax seeds, and lemon juice until smooth.

Silky Strawberry Smoothie

Preparation Time: 10 minutes
Cooking Time: 15 minutes
Servings: 1

Ingredients:
- 1 cup fresh strawberries
- One banana, sliced
- 1 cup ice
- ½ cup silken tofu
- One teaspoon of agave nectar (optional)

Directions:
- ➢ Combine strawberries, banana, rice, tofu, and agave nectar in a blender until smooth.

Fruit Smoothie II

Preparation Time: 10 minutes
Cooking Time: 15 minutes
Servings: 1

Ingredients:
- 1 cup blueberries
- Two apples - peeled, cored and chopped
- 1 ½ cups raspberries
- ¾ cup seedless grapes
- Three tablespoons of white sugar
- One tray of ice cubes

Directions:
- ➢ Combine blueberries, apples, raspberries, grapes, sugar, and ice in a blender. Blend until completely smooth. Pour into serving glasses and serve.

Raspberry and Apricot Smoothie

Preparation Time: 10 minutes
Cooking Time: 15 minutes
Servings: 1

Ingredients:

- ¾ cup raspberries, or to taste
- ½ cup plain fat-free Greek yoghurt
- ½ cup crushed ice
- One apricot - peeled, pitted, and chopped
- Two tablespoons honey
- One tablespoon of flax seeds
- One tablespoon of lemon juice

Directions:
- ➢ Blend raspberries, yoghurt, ice, apricot, honey, flax seeds, and lemon juice together in a blender until smooth.

Holly Goodness Smoothie

Preparation Time: 10 minutes
Cooking Time: 15 minutes
Servings: 1

Ingredients:
- One mango - peeled, seeded, and chopped
- One small banana
- ½ cup frozen raspberries
- ½ cup almond milk
- ½ cup hemp milk
- One teaspoon of vanilla extract
- One teaspoon of chia seeds
- One teaspoon of hemp seeds
- One teaspoon of maca powder

Directions:
- ➢ In a blender, combine mango, banana, raspberries, almond milk, hemp milk, vanilla essence, chia seeds, hemp seeds, and maca powder until smooth.

Breakfast Power Smoothie

Preparation Time: 10 minutes
Cooking Time: 15 minutes
Servings: 1

Ingredients:
- 1 cup So Delicious® Dairy Free Unsweetened Coconutmilk Beverage
- Two bananas, peeled and frozen
- 1 ½ cup frozen strawberries
- One packet of vanilla protein powder (such as Vega One French Vanilla)
- 1 cup chopped kale or spinach (optional)

Directions:
- ➢ In a blender, combine all of the ingredients.
- ➢ Blend until completely smooth. Enjoy!

CHAPTER 10: BREAKFAST

Breakfast Apples

Preparation Time: 10 minutes
Cooking Time: 15 minutes
Servings: 1

Ingredients:

- One apple, cored and chopped
- ½ cup crispy rice cereal squares (such as Rice Chex®), crushed
- Two teaspoons of ground cinnamon
- Two teaspoons of coconut oil
- ½ cup sliced fresh strawberries (optional)
- ¼ cup chopped walnuts (optional)

Directions:

➢ Combine the apple, rice cereal, cinnamon, and coconut oil in a microwave-safe bowl.
➢ Microwave for 30 to 45 seconds or until the coconut oil is melted. To blend, stir everything together.
➢ If preferred, top with berries and walnuts.

Venison Breakfast Sausage

Preparation Time: 10 minutes
Cooking Time: 15 minutes
Servings: 1

Ingredients:

- 1 pound ground venison
- 8 ounces bacon, minced
- One teaspoon of ground sage
- ½ teaspoon ground ginger
- ¼ teaspoon pepper
- ¾ teaspoon onion salt

Directions:

➢ Combine the venison, bacon, sage, ginger, pepper, and onion salt in a large mixing bowl. Form the mixture into 12 patties, about 1/4 cup of each burger. Patties can be cooked in a skillet or frozen for later use.

Breakfast Brownies

Preparation Time: 10 minutes
Cooking Time: 15 minutes
Servings: 1

Ingredients:

- 1 ½ cups quick-cooking oats
- ¾ cup brown sugar
- ¾ cup flax seed meal
- ½ cup gluten-free all-purpose baking flour
- One teaspoon of baking powder
- ½ teaspoon ground cinnamon
- ¼ teaspoon salt
- One banana, mashed
- ¼ cup rice milk
- One egg
- One teaspoon of vanilla extract

Directions:

➢ Preheat the oven carefully carefully to 350°F (175 degrees C). Grease an 8x10-inch baking pan lightly.
➢ Combine oats, brown sugar, flax seed meal, flour, baking powder, cinnamon, and salt in a mixing basin. Combine the banana, rice milk, egg, and vanilla essence in a separate dish. Stir the banana mixture into the flour mixture. Fill the prepared baking pan halfway with batter.
➢ Bake the brownies for 20 minutes, or until a toothpick inserted into the middle comes out clean. Cover the pan with a cloth to keep the moisture in and allow the brownies to cool for at least 5 minutes before serving.

Susie's Breakfast Casserole

Preparation Time: 10 minutes
Cooking Time: 15 minutes
Servings: 1

Ingredients:

- Six eggs, beaten
- 1 cup milk
- ½ teaspoon salt
- ⅛ teaspoon ground black pepper
- cooking spray
- Three slices of bread, torn into pieces
- 1 (12 ounces) package of cooked breakfast sausage
- ½ cup Monterey Jack cheese
- ½ cup shredded Cheddar cheese

Directions:

➢ Combine the eggs, milk, salt, and black pepper in a mixing dish.
➢ Coat a 2-quart baking dish with nonstick cooking spray. Spread an even layer of bread on the bottom of the prepared dish; top with sausage, Monterey Jack cheese, egg mixture, then Cheddar cheese, in that order. Refrigerate the baking dish, covered with plastic wrap, for 8 hours overnight.
➢ Preheat the oven carefully to 325°F (165 degrees C). Remove dish from refrigerator and set aside for 15 minutes to come to room temperature.
➢ Bake the casserole in a preheated oven for 45 minutes or until it is bubbling and hot.

Breakfast Cheesesteaks

Preparation Time: 10 minutes
Cooking Time: 15 minutes
Servings: 1

Ingredients:

- Six large eggs, divided
- Two tablespoons milk
- Four thick slices of bread
- 1 (5 ounces) package Jones Dairy Farm All Natural Golden Brown® Chicken Sausage Patties
- One tablespoon of olive oil
- One clove of garlic, minced
- ½ red bell pepper, thinly sliced
- ½ green bell pepper, thinly sliced
- ½ small red onion, thinly sliced
- 2 slices provolone cheese
- Salt and pepper to taste

Directions:

➢ Combine two eggs and milk in a medium mixing dish; dip bread into the egg mixture until completely covered. Cook French toast until golden brown on both sides on a grill or big pan over medium heat.
➢ Cook the sausage patties according to the package directions. Make strips out of it.
➢ Warm the olive oil in a separate skillet over medium heat. Sauté the garlic, peppers, and onions until browned and tender.
➢ Cook until the cheese is melted, then add the cooked sausage slices to the pepper and onion combination.
➢ Cook the remaining eggs over easy or to your liking.

➤ Layer french toast with eggs, pepper, sausage, and cheese mixture, then top with cheesesteaks. Serve open-faced with salt and pepper.

Breakfast Crisp

Preparation Time: 10 minutes
Cooking Time: 15 minutes
Servings: 1

Ingredients:
- 1 ½ cups quick-cooking oats
- ½ cup unbleached all-purpose flour
- One teaspoon of baking powder
- ½ teaspoon ground cinnamon
- ½ teaspoon salt
- ½ cup brown sugar
- ¼ cup margarine softened
- One egg

Directions:
➤ Preheat the oven carefully to 350°F (175 degrees C). Grease a 9x9-inch baking pan lightly.
➤ Combine the oats, flour, baking powder, cinnamon, and salt in a large mixing basin. Cream together brown sugar and margarine in a separate dish. Incorporate the egg. Stir the contents together just until combined. Pour the batter into the prepared pan.
➤ Bake for 30 minutes, or until a toothpick inserted into the middle of the pan comes out clean.

Easy Breakfast Pizzas

Preparation Time: 10 minutes
Cooking Time: 15 minutes
Servings: 1

Ingredients:
- Five plain bagels, split
- 1 (14 ounces) package of cooked bacon, cut into 1/4-inch pieces
- 1 cup prepared sausage gravy
- 1 (8 ounces) package of shredded mozzarella cheese

Directions:
➤ Preheat the oven carefully to 350°F (175 degrees C).
➤ Place the bagels on a baking pan, and cut sides up. Arrange the bacon slices on top of the bagel halves. Lightly spoon gravy on top of the bacon. Over the gravy, sprinkle with mozzarella cheese.
➤ Bake for about 10 minutes or until the cheese melts.

Low-Fat Breakfast Muffins

Preparation Time: 10 minutes
Cooking Time: 15 minutes
Servings: 1

Ingredients:
- cooking spray
- 2 cups multigrain toasted oat cereal (such as Cheerios®)
- One ¼ cup all-purpose flour
- ¼ cup brown sugar
- One teaspoon of baking powder
- ¾ teaspoon baking soda
- 1 cup mashed bananas
- ⅔ cup skim milk
- Two egg whites
- ¼ cup unsweetened applesauce
- ¼ cup raisins
- ¼ cup semisweet chocolate chips (Optional)

Directions:
➤ Preheat the oven carefully to 400° F. (200 degrees C). Cooking spray should be used to grease 12 standard muffin cups.

➤ Fill a resealable plastic bag halfway with cereal. 1 1/2 cups crushed gently with a rolling pin
➤ Combine crushed cereal, flour, brown sugar, baking powder, and baking soda in a large mixing basin. Add mashed bananas, milk, egg whites, applesauce, raisins, and chocolate chips until barely moistened. Divide the batter evenly between the muffin cups.
➤ 18 to 22 minutes in a preheated oven until golden brown. Allow for 2 minutes in the pan before transferring to a cooling rack. If preferred, serve warm.

Breakfast Pizza I

Preparation Time: 10 minutes
Cooking Time: 15 minutes
Servings: 1

Ingredients:
- 1 pound ground breakfast sausage
- 1 (8 ounces) package of refrigerated crescent rolls
- 1 cup frozen hash brown potatoes, thawed
- 1 cup shredded Cheddar cheese
- Five eggs
- ¼ cup milk
- ½ teaspoon salt
- ⅛ teaspoon ground black pepper
- ¼ cup grated Parmesan cheese

Directions:
➤ In a big, deep-pan, brown the sausage. Cook until uniformly browned over medium-high heat. Set aside after draining and crumbling. Preheat the oven carefully to 375°F (190 degrees C).
➤ Brown the sausage and drain it. Make eight triangles out of the crescent roll dough. Place in a 12-inch ungreased pizza pan with the tips toward the middle. Form a crust by pressing the ingredients together. The bottom of the crust should be sealed, and the outside border should be elevated slightly. Spread the sausage over the crust. Serve with hash browns and cheddar cheese on top.
➤ Combine eggs, milk, salt, and pepper in a mixing bowl; pour over crust—season with parmesan cheese.
➤ Bake in a preheated oven for 25 to 30 minutes, or until the eggs are set.

Breakfast Pasta

Preparation Time: 10 minutes
Cooking Time: 15 minutes
Servings: 1

Ingredients:
- ½ (14 ounces) package of spaghetti
- Three tablespoons of olive oil, divided
- Four eggs, beaten
- ½ onion, diced
- ¼ cup chopped baby Bella (crimini) mushrooms
- ¼ cup frozen peas
- ¼ cup shredded carrots
- ½ cup freshly grated Parmesan cheese
- salt and ground black pepper to taste

Directions:
➤ Warm up a big saucepan of gently salted water. Cook the spaghetti in boiling water for 12 minutes, tossing periodically, until cooked through yet firm to the biting. Drain.
➤ Heat one tablespoon of oil in a pan over medium heat; cook and whisk eggs in the heated oil until set and scrambled for about 5 minutes.
➤ In a separate pan, heat the remaining two tablespoons of oil over medium-high heat and sauté the onion, mushrooms, peas, and carrots until the onion is caramelized, about 10 minutes. Toss the spaghetti with the onion mixture. Mix in the eggs well. Toss the spaghetti with the Parmesan cheese, salt, and pepper.

Sweet Potato Breakfast Bake

Preparation Time: 10 minutes
Cooking Time: 15 minutes
Servings: 1

Ingredients:
- One tablespoon of olive oil
- One sweet potato, diced
- 1 pound sausage
- ½ cup chopped onion
- ½ red bell pepper, diced
- 1 cup sliced fresh mushrooms
- 1 cup torn kale leaves
- salt and ground black pepper to taste
- Five eggs
- ⅓ cup water
- One teaspoon of dried thyme, or to taste
- One green onion, diced

Directions:
- ➢ Preheat the oven carefully to 400°F (200 degrees C).
- ➢ In a large pan over medium heat, heat the olive oil. Cover and boil, occasionally stirring, until sweet potato is cooked for 8 to 10 minutes. Transfer to a large mixing bowl.
- ➢ Cook and stir sausage in the same pan over medium-high heat for 5 minutes, or until crumbled and browned. Combine with the sweet potato in the bowl.
- ➢ Cook and toss the onion and red bell pepper in the same pan until about 3 minutes. Season with salt and pepper to taste. Cook until the mushrooms and greens soften, approximately 3 minutes longer. Transfer to a mixing basin.
- ➢ Combine the eggs, water, thyme, salt, and pepper in a small mixing dish. Combine with the sausage mixture. Fill a large baking dish halfway with the mixture.
- ➢ Bake for 20 to 25 minutes, or until the sweet potato begins to colour. Allow standing for 5 minutes. Garnish with green onion if desired.

Perfect Breakfast

Preparation Time: 10 minutes
Cooking Time: 15 minutes
Servings: 1

Ingredients:
- Two teaspoons butter
- Two eggs
- One slice of sourdough bread, toasted
- Dijon mustard
- ½ avocado - peeled, pitted, and sliced
- Two tablespoons grated Parmesan cheese, or more to taste

Directions:
- ➢ In a pan over medium heat, melt two tablespoons of butter; add the eggs. Allow the egg whites to cook until mostly hard before breaking in the yolks; simmer until the eggs are cooked and no longer runny, 2 to 3 minutes.
- ➢ Dijon mustard on one side of a toasted sourdough bread piece
- ➢ Arrange the avocado slices on top of the mustard.
- ➢ Cooked eggs should be placed on top of the avocado.
- ➢ Sprinkle Parmesan cheese on top of the eggs.

Chorizo Breakfast Burritos

Preparation Time: 10 minutes
Cooking Time: 15 minutes
Servings: 1

Ingredients:
- cooking spray
- ¾ pound chorizo sausage, casings removed and crumbled
- ½ cup chopped red onion
- One green chile pepper, seeded and diced
- Four eggs
- Four flour tortillas
- 1 cup shredded Cheddar cheese

Directions:
- ➢ Coat a big frying pan liberally with cooking spray. Cook and stir chorizo until fully browned and crumbled over medium-high heat. Continue cooking until the onion and chile pepper is soft.
- ➢ In a separate dish, whisk the eggs and add them to the chorizo mixture. Reduce the heat to medium-low and continue to cook, constantly stirring, until the eggs are scrambled and no longer runny.
- ➢ Microwave the flour tortillas for 30 seconds. Fill each tortilla with the mixture and top with grated Cheddar cheese. Roll it up like a tortilla and eat it!

Sausage Breakfast Casserole

Preparation Time: 10 minutes
Cooking Time: 15 minutes
Servings: 1

Ingredients:
- 1 (16 ounces) package bulk breakfast sausage
- One green onion, chopped
- 1 (16 ounces) package of hash brown potatoes
- 2 cups shredded Cheddar cheese
- Six large eggs, lightly beaten
- 1 cup milk
- 1 (2.64 ounces) package of country gravy mix
- One pinch of ground paprika, or to taste

Directions:
- ➢ Preheat the oven carefully to 325° F. (165 degrees C). Grease an 8x11-inch baking dish with cooking spray.
- ➢ Cook and stir breakfast sausage in a pan over medium heat for 10 minutes, or until browned and crumbled; drain excess fat.
- ➢ Mix the green onion with the sausage and distribute it in the prepared baking dish. Spread a layer of hash brown potatoes on top, then sprinkle with Cheddar cheese.
- ➢ In a mixing basin, combine eggs, milk, and gravy mix until combined; pour over a casserole—season with paprika to taste.
- ➢ Bake for 1 hour, or until a knife inserted into the middle of the dish comes out clean. Allow standing for 10 minutes before serving to firm up.

Black Bean Breakfast Bowl

Preparation Time: 10 minutes
Cooking Time: 15 minutes
Servings: 1

Ingredients:
- Two tablespoons of olive oil
- Four eggs, beaten
- 1 can of black beans, drained and rinsed
- One avocado, peeled and sliced
- ¼ cup salsa
- salt and ground black pepper to taste

Directions:
- ➢ In a small saucepan over medium heat, heat the olive oil. Cook and whisk eggs for 3 to 5 minutes or until they are set.
- ➢ Fill a microwave-safe dish halfway with black beans—microwave on High for 1 minute, or until heated.
- ➢ Divide the warmed black beans across two dishes.
- ➢ Scrambled eggs, avocado, and salsa should be added to each bowl—season with salt and black pepper to taste.

Low Fat Breakfast Cookies

Preparation Time: 10 minutes
Cooking Time: 15 minutes
Servings: 1

Ingredients:

- 1 ½ cup rolled oats
- ½ cup whole wheat flour
- ½ cup all-purpose flour
- ½ cup light brown sugar
- 1 ½ teaspoon wheat germ
- ½ teaspoon baking powder
- ½ teaspoon baking soda
- ¼ teaspoon salt
- One ripe banana, mashed
- ¼ cup unsweetened applesauce
- Two egg whites
- One teaspoon of vanilla extract
- ½ cup chocolate chips
- ½ cup dried cranberries

Directions:
- ➤ Preheat the oven carefully to 350°F (175 degrees C). Use parchment paper or a silicone mat to line a baking sheet.
- ➤ In a large mixing bowl, combine oats, whole wheat flour, all-purpose flour, brown sugar, wheat germ, baking powder, baking soda, and salt. Mix in the banana, applesauce, egg whites, and vanilla essence. Fold in the chocolate chips and cranberries gently. One spoonful at a time, drop batter onto a prepared baking sheet.
- ➤ Bake for 12 minutes in a preheated oven until golden brown.

Richard's Breakfast Scramble

Preparation Time: 10 minutes
Cooking Time: 15 minutes
Servings: 1

Ingredients:
- Five eggs, beaten
- Two tablespoons milk
- 1 cup shredded Cheddar cheese
- One onion, chopped
- Two slices of cooked ham
- ⅛ teaspoon garlic powder
- 1 to taste salt and pepper
- 2 ½ tablespoons butter

Directions:
- ➤ In a large mixing basin, combine eggs and milk. Combine the onion, ham, cheese, salt, pepper, and garlic powder in a mixing bowl.
- ➤ Melt the butter in a large frying pan or skillet over medium-high heat. Cook, without stirring until the eggs begin to set. Stir the eggs until they are fairly scrambled. Continue doing this for 10 to 15 minutes, or until the eggs are thoroughly cooked. Serve hot.

Breakfast Power Smoothie

Preparation Time: 10 minutes
Cooking Time: 15 minutes
Servings: 1

Ingredients:
- cup So Delicious® Dairy Free Unsweetened Coconutmilk Beverage
- Two bananas, peeled and frozen
- 1 ½ cup frozen strawberries

- One packet of vanilla protein powder (such as Vega One French Vanilla)
- 1 cup chopped kale or spinach (optional)

Directions:
- ➤ In a blender, combine all of the ingredients.
- ➤ Blend until completely smooth. Enjoy!

Best Breakfast Quesadilla

Preparation Time: 10 minutes
Cooking Time: 15 minutes
Servings: 1

Ingredients:
- Two large eggs
- Three slices of bacon, cooked and crumbled
- 2 (8 inches) flour tortillas
- One teaspoon butter, softened, or to taste
- cooking spray
- ½ cup shredded Colby-Jack cheese

Directions:
- ➤ In a small dish, crack the eggs. Whisk in the crumbled bacon until thoroughly mixed.
- ➤ Coat a big skillet with cooking spray and heat on medium-high. Pour egg mixture into skillet; heat and stir for 5 minutes, or until eggs are set. Take the pan off the heat.
- ➤ Butter one side of each tortilla lightly.
- ➤ Warm a dry skillet over medium-low heat in a separate pan.
- ➤ Place one tortilla in the heated skillet, greased side down. The side of the scrambled egg mixture should be spread over one half of the tortilla. Fold the tortilla over the egg mixture and top with 1/4 cup Colby-Jack cheese. Cook, occasionally flipping, for 2 to 3 minutes, or until the tortilla is toasted and crispy and the cheese is melted. Rep to create the second quesadilla.

Breakfast Sausage

Preparation Time: 10 minutes
Cooking Time: 15 minutes
Servings: 1

Ingredients:
- One tablespoon of brown sugar
- Two teaspoons of dried sage
- Two teaspoons salt
- One teaspoon of ground black pepper
- ¼ teaspoon dried marjoram
- ⅛ teaspoon crushed red pepper flakes
- One pinch of ground cloves
- 2 pounds of ground pork

Directions:
- ➤ Add brown sugar, sage, salt, black pepper, marjoram, red pepper flakes, and cloves to a small mixing dish.
- ➤ Pork should be placed in a large mixing dish. Mix in the spice mixture with your hands until fully blended. Make six patties out of the mixture.
- ➤ Melt butter in a large pan over medium-high heat. Cook until the patties are golden and crispy, about 5 minutes per side. In the middle, an instant-read thermometer should read at least 160 degrees F. (71 degrees C).

CHAPTER 11: STEWS & SOUPS

Baked Corn Tortilla Strips for Mexican Soups
Preparation Time: 10 minutes
Cooking Time: 15 minutes
Servings: 1

Ingredients:
- 8 (6 inches) corn tortillas
- Two tablespoons avocado oil, or more as needed

Directions:
- ➢ Preheat the oven carefully to 350° F. (175 degrees C).
- ➢ Tortillas should be cut in half first, then crosswise into 1/8-inch strips. Toss in a dish with oil until evenly coated. Arrange tortilla strips on a baking sheet in a single layer.
- ➢ Bake for 15 minutes, or until the strips are crisp and gently browned. Remove from the oven and set aside to cool.

Fabulous Roasted Cauliflower Soup
Preparation Time: 10 minutes
Cooking Time: 15 minutes
Servings: 1

Ingredients:
- Two heads of cauliflower, separated into florets
- Threehree cloves of garlic, chopped
- Two shallots, chopped
- One tablespoon of olive oil
- 3 cups chicken broth
- 1 cup water
- One bay learned
- One teaspoon of dried thyme
- 2 cups heavy cream
- salt and pepper

Directions:
- ➢ Preheat the oven carefully to 425° F. (220 degrees C). Toss cauliflower with olive oil, garlic, and shallots in a large mixing basin. Spread out on a baking sheet or roasting pan with edges.
- ➢ Thirtyirty minutes in a preheated oven until browned and tender.
- ➢ Transfer the cauliflower to a soup pot and add the chicken stock and water. Bring to a boil, season with thyme and bay leaf, and serve—Cook for 30 minutes on medium heat. Remove the bay leaf and set it aside.
- ➢ Use an immersion blender to puree the soup in the pot, or transfer to a blender and purée in stages before returning to the pot—season with salt and pepper after adding the cream. Before serving, heat thoroughly but do not boil.

Slow Cooker Fresh Vegetable-Beef-Barley Soup
Preparation Time: 10 minutes
Cooking Time: 15 minutes
Servings: 1

Ingredients:
- 1 ½ pound cubed beef stew meat
- 2 (14.5 ounces) cans of diced tomatoes with garlic
- 1 (12 ounces) can tomato-vegetable juice cocktail (such as V8®)
- Two large potatoes, diced
- 1 (8 ounces) can of tomato sauce
- 1 cup sliced carrot
- ¾ cup barley
- ¾ cup chopped onion
- ¾ cup frozen green beans
- ½ cup chopped bell pepper
- ⅔ cup frozen whole kernel corn
- ½ cup chopped celery
- One tablespoon of Worcestershire sauce
- ½ teaspoon dried parsley
- ¼ teaspoon ground thyme
- ¼ teaspoon dried oregano
- ¼ teaspoon dried marjoram
- ¼ teaspoon dried basil
- Two beef bouillon cubes
- sea salt and ground black pepper
- Two bay leaves
- 2 cups sliced fresh mushrooms

Directions:
- ➢ In the crock of a large slow cooker, combine beef, diced tomatoes with garlic, tomato-vegetable juice cocktail, potatoes, tomato sauce, carrot green beans, corn, bell pepper, celery, barley, onion, Worcestershire sauce, parsley, thyme, oregano, marjoram, basil, beef bouillon cubes, bay leaves, sea salt, and black pepper.
- ➢ Cook on Low for 7 to 8 hours, or until the meat is tender. Cook for another hour after adding the mushrooms.

Potato Soup
Preparation Time: 10 minutes
Cooking Time: 15 minutes
Servings: 1

Ingredients:
- One tablespoon butter
- One large onion, chopped
- 6 cups mashed cooked potatoes
- 2 (14.5 ounces) can chicken broth
- ½ cup milk

Directions:
- ➢ Melt butter in a medium soup pot over low heat and sauté onions until soft. Stir in the mashed potatoes, followed by the chicken broth. Add milk while stirring (use more or less to achieve desired creaminess). Cook until well cooked, then season with salt & pepper to taste.

Fennel Soup
Preparation Time: 10 minutes
Cooking Time: 15 minutes
Servings: 1

Ingredients:
- ¼ cup butter
- Five fennel bulbs, trimmed and quartered
- 1 (32 fluid ounce) container of vegetable broth
- salt and pepper to taste

Directions:
- ➢ In a large pan over medium heat, melt the butter. Cook and stir until the fennel bulbs are golden brown, about 10 minutes. Pour in the stock and cook for another 15 minutes, or until the fennel is soft—season with salt and pepper before ladling into soup cups.

Leek and Fennel Soup
Preparation Time: 10 minutes
Cooking Time: 15 minutes
Servings: 1

Ingredients:

- Two tablespoons of olive oil
- Three large leeks, cleaned and thinly sliced
- Four large stalks of celery, thinly sliced
- Three large white onions, peeled and halved
- One large fennel bulb, thinly sliced
- Two large baking potatoes
- One tablespoon salt
- 1 ½ teaspoon ground black pepper
- 8 cups water
- 2 cubes vegetable bouillon

Directions:

- ➤ Cook and whisk the olive oil, leeks, celery, onions, fennel, potatoes, salt, and pepper in a large saucepan or soup kettle over medium-low heat until the onions are translucent and the vegetables have begun to soften, approximately 10 minutes.
- ➤ Bring 8 cups of water to a boil over the veggies, decrease the heat and add the vegetable bouillon cubes. Simmer, stirring periodically to dissolve the cubes, for 30 minutes, or until the vegetables are soft and the potatoes have begun to thicken the soup.

Oxtail Soup I

Preparation Time: 10 minutes
Cooking Time: 15 minutes
Servings: 1

Ingredients:

- 3 pounds beef oxtail
- Three teaspoons salt
- ¼ teaspoon ground black pepper
- One onion, chopped
- Two carrots, sliced
- One parsnip, sliced
- One turnip, peeled and diced
- Two tablespoons of brandy (Optional)
- 6 cups water
- ½ teaspoon dried savoury
- One bay leaf
- ½ cup barley
- 2 ounces dried mushrooms

Directions:

- ➤ For 30 to 45 minutes, soak dried mushrooms in boiling water. Drain and cut into slices.
- ➤ Remove all fat from the oxtails. Spread the mixture in a shallow roasting pan. Forty-five minutes at 450 degrees F (230 degrees C). Reserve roughly two tablespoons of the fat.
- ➤ One cup of water should be added to the roasting pan where the oxtails were browned. Stir regularly while heating to dissolve the browned bits. Reserve.
- ➤ Sauté onion, carrots, parsnip, mushrooms, and turnip in conserved fat until tender, about 10 minutes. Brown the oxtails—drizzle brandy over the sautéed vegetables. Ignite.
- ➤ Pour the oxtails and veggies with the conserved water and brown. Pour in the remaining 5 cups of water: Savoury, bay leaf, barley, salt, and pepper to taste. Bring to a boil, then turn down the heat. Cover and simmer for 2 hours on low heat—season to taste.

Cold Cucumber Soup

Preparation Time: 10 minutes
Cooking Time: 15 minutes
Servings: 1

Ingredients:

- 16 ounces plain whole-milk yoghurt
- Two large cucumbers
- One ⅓ cups buttermilk
- ¼ cup finely chopped fresh mint

- One small bunch of chopped fresh flat-leaf parsley, or to taste
- Two cloves garlic
- One tablespoon of extra virgin olive oil
- salt and ground white pepper to taste

Directions:

- ➤ Line a fine sieve with cheesecloth or a coffee filter. After 30 minutes, filter the yoghurt. Pour away any accumulated whey.
- ➤ Cucumbers should be peeled; the seeds should be scraped out and discarded. Place cucumber in a blender and roughly chop—puree 1/2 of the yoghurt, 1/2 of the buttermilk, and one garlic clove. Process the remaining yoghurt, buttermilk, garlic, mint, and parsley until everything is finely blended. Depending on the size of your blender, you may need to work in batches—season with salt and pepper and drizzle with olive oil.

Cream of Fresh Tomato Soup

Preparation Time: 10 minutes
Cooking Time: 15 minutes
Servings: 1

Ingredients:

- Two large tomatoes, chopped
- ½ cup chopped onion
- ½ teaspoon white sugar
- salt to taste
- ground black pepper to taste
- Two tablespoons margarine
- Two tablespoons of all-purpose flour
- 2 cups milk

Directions:

- ➤ Cook tomatoes, onions, sugar, salt, and pepper in a saucepan. When the onions are tender, strain them. Set aside the liquid.
- ➤ Melt the butter or margarine in a saucepan. Incorporate the flour. Cook until the milk has thickened, whisking constantly. Slowly pour in the saved tomato juice and heat gradually. Serve immediately.

Basic Chicken Stock

Preparation Time: 10 minutes
Cooking Time: 15 minutes
Servings: 1

Ingredients:

- 1 pound of chicken parts
- One large onion
- Three stalks of celery, including some leaves
- One large carrot
- 1 ½ teaspoons salt
- Three whole cloves
- 6 cups water (Optional)
- ¼ cup cold water (Optional)
- One egg

Directions:

- ➤ Cut onion into quarters. One-inch slices of cleaned celery and carrot combine the chicken, onion, celery, carrot, salt, and cloves in a large soup pot or Dutch oven—six cups of water. Bring the water to a boil. Reduce the heat to low, cover, and leave to simmer for 1 hour.
- ➤ Take out the chicken and veggies. The stock should be strained. Remove the fat off the surface.
- ➤ Follow this procedure to clarify stock for clear soup, eliminating solid specks that are too fine to drain out using cheesecloth. Separate the egg white from the yolk, keeping the shell aside. 1/4 cup cold water, egg white, and broken eggshell in a small basin. Bring to a boil with the strained stock. Remove from the heat and set aside for 5 minutes. Again, strain through a cheesecloth-lined sieve.

Homemade Vegetable Beef Soup

Preparation Time: 10 minutes
Cooking Time: 15 minutes
Servings: 1

Ingredients:

- 1 ½ pound beef stew meat, cut into 1/2-inch cubes
- 2 (14 ounces) can beef broth
- 1 (15 ounces) can of green beans, drained
- 1 can of whole kernel corn, drained
- 1 (14.5 ounces) can of tomato sauce
- 1 (6 ounces) can of tomato paste
- 1 (46 fluid ounce) bottle tomato-vegetable juice cocktail (such as V8®)
- ¼ teaspoon garlic powder, or to taste
- ¼ tablespoon onion powder, or to taste
- salt and ground black pepper, to taste

Directions:

➤ Combine beef broth and beef stew meat in a large saucepan over medium heat. Bring broth to a boil, lower to low heat and cook meat until tender, about 45 minutes.
➤ Combine the meat, corn, green beans, tomato sauce, and tomato paste in a mixing bowl. Season the tomato-vegetable juice cocktail with garlic powder, onion powder, salt, and pepper. Bring the mixture to a boil, then lower to low heat for 5 hours.

Steak Soup

Preparation Time: 10 minutes
Cooking Time: 15 minutes
Servings: 1

Ingredients:

- Two tablespoons butter
- Two tablespoons of vegetable oil
- 1 ½ pound lean boneless beef round steak, cut into cubes
- ½ cup chopped onion
- Three tablespoons of all-purpose flour
- One tablespoon paprika
- One teaspoon salt
- ¼ teaspoon ground black pepper
- 4 cups beef broth
- 2 cups water
- Four sprigs of fresh parsley, chopped
- Two tablespoons of chopped celery leaves
- One bay leaf
- ½ teaspoon dried marjoram
- 1 ½ cups peeled, diced Yukon Gold potatoes
- 1 ½ cup sliced carrots
- 1 ½ cups chopped celery
- 1 (6 ounces) can of tomato paste
- 1 can of whole kernel corn

Directions:

➤ Melt the butter and oil in a large pan over medium heat until the foam from the butter evaporates, then add the steak pieces and onion—Cook and stir for 10 minutes, or until the meat and onion are browned. While the meat is cooking, combine the flour, paprika, salt, and pepper in a mixing bowl. To coat, sprinkle the flour mixture over the browned meat.
➤ Pour the beef broth and water into a large soup pot and whisk in the parsley, celery leaves, bay leaf, and marjoram. Bring to a boil with the meat mixture. Reduce the heat to medium-low, cover the pot, and simmer for 45 minutes until the meat is cooked.
➤ Stir in the potatoes, carrots, celery, tomato paste, and corn; return the soup to a boil and cook, uncovered, for 15 to 20 minutes, or until the vegetables are soft and the soup is thick. Remove the bay leaf and serve immediately.

Chicken and Gnocchi Soup

Preparation Time: 10 minutes
Cooking Time: 15 minutes
Servings: 1

Ingredients:

- One tablespoon of olive oil
- One small onion, diced
- Three stalks of celery, diced
- Three cloves of garlic, minced
- Two carrots, shredded
- 1 pound cooked, cubed chicken breast
- 4 cups chicken broth
- 1 (16 ounces) package of mini potato gnocchi
- 1 (6 ounces) bag of baby spinach leaves
- One tablespoon cornstarch (Optional)
- Two tablespoons of cold water (Optional)
- 2 cups half-and-half cream
- salt and ground black pepper to taste

Directions:

➤ In a large saucepan, heat the olive oil over medium heat. Cook the onion, celery, garlic, and carrots in the heated oil for 5 minutes or until the onion is transparent. Bring to a boil with the cubed chicken and chicken broth.
➤ Cook until the gnocchi begins to float in the boiling broth, 3 to 4 minutes. Cook until the spinach is wilted, about 3 minutes more.
➤ Until smooth, whisk cornstarch into cold water. Stir the cornstarch/half-and-half mixture into the boiling soup. Cook for 5 minutes, or until the soup thickens slightly. Season with salt and black pepper to taste.

Chicken Vegetable Barley Soup

Preparation Time: 10 minutes
Cooking Time: 15 minutes
Servings: 1

Ingredients:

- 1 cup slivered almonds
- Two tablespoons of olive oil
- One medium onion, chopped
- 1 cup chopped celery
- 4 cups sliced fresh mushrooms
- Four cloves of garlic, minced
- 1 cup chopped carrots
- 5 cups diced red potatoes
- 3 cups chopped cooked chicken
- 2 ½ quarts of chicken broth
- 1 cup quick-cooking barley
- Two tablespoons butter
- ½ cup chopped fresh parsley
- salt and black pepper to taste

Directions:

➤ Preheat the oven carefully to 400°F (200 degrees C). A baking sheet should be equally covered with slivered almonds. Toast till golden brown and aromatic in a preheated oven.
➤ In a large stockpot over medium heat, heat the oil. Cook until the onions, celery, mushrooms, and garlic are soft in oil.
➤ Combine carrots, potatoes, chicken, and broth in a mixing bowl. Bring to a boil before stirring in the barley. Reduce the heat to low, cover, and cook for 20 minutes.
➤ Take the pan off the heat and whisk in the butter, parsley, and toasted almonds—season to taste with salt and pepper.

Ground Turkey Soup with Beans

Preparation Time: 10 minutes
Cooking Time: 15 minutes
Servings: 1

Ingredients:
- 2 pounds of ground turkey
- 12 medium (blank)s baby carrots, finely chopped
- One medium onion, chopped
- Four stalks of celery, chopped
- Four medium red potatoes, cut into 1-inch pieces
- 1 (15 ounces) can of tomato sauce
- 1 (15 ounces) can of whole peeled tomatoes, crushed
- 1 (15 ounces) can of peas, undrained
- 1 (15 ounces) can of green beans, drained and rinsed
- 1 (15 ounces) can of kidney beans, rinsed and drained
- 1 can of whole kernel corn
- ground black pepper to taste
- One pinch of seasoned salt (such as Morton® Nature's Seasons® Seasoning Blend), or to taste
- One pinch of ground thyme
- One bay leaf or more to taste
- 1 cup water, or more to taste

Directions:
- ➢ In a stockpot over medium-high heat, crumble the turkey. Cook and stir for 7 to 10 minutes, or until uniformly browned, crumbly, and no longer pink. Any surplus grease should be drained and discarded.
- ➢ Cook and whisk in the carrots, onion, and celery until the veggies are tender, about 5 minutes. Potatoes, tomato sauce, tomatoes, undrained peas, green beans, kidney beans, and corn are good additions—season with black pepper and seasoned salt to taste. Stir until everything is uniformly distributed. Mix in the thyme and bay leaf.
- ➢ Bring the water to a simmer in the saucepan. Cook, covered, for 1 hour, stirring frequently and adding extra water as required, until potatoes are soft.

Cream of Asparagus Soup I
Preparation Time: 10 minutes
Cooking Time: 15 minutes
Servings: 1

Ingredients:
- ¼ cup margarine
- One onion, chopped
- Three stalks of celery, chopped
- Three tablespoons of all-purpose flour
- 4 cups water
- 1 (10.5 ounces) can of condensed chicken broth
- Four tablespoons of chicken bouillon powder
- One potato, peeled and diced
- 1 pound fresh asparagus, trimmed and coarsely chopped
- ¾ cup half-and-half
- One tablespoon of soy sauce
- ¼ teaspoon ground black pepper
- ¼ teaspoon ground white pepper

Directions:
- ➢ In a heavy saucepan, melt the butter or margarine. Cook until the onions and celery are soft, approximately 4 minutes. Mix in the flour well. Cook, stirring regularly, for approximately 1 minute. Do not allow it to burn or get lumpy. Stir in the water, chicken broth, and chicken soup base until smooth. Bring the water to a boil. Toss in the diced potatoes and asparagus. Simmer for around 20 minutes on low heat.
- ➢ In batches, puree the soup in a food processor or blender. Return to the pot.
- ➢ Add the half-and-half cream, soy sauce, and black and white pepper to taste. Bring soup to a boil. Seasonings can be adjusted to taste. Serve immediately.

Best Butternut Squash Soup Ever
Preparation Time: 10 minutes
Cooking Time: 15 minutes

Servings: 1

Ingredients:
- 1 ½ tablespoons butter
- ½ onion, sliced
- Two cloves garlic
- Two sprigs of fresh thyme
- ½ butternut squash - peeled, seeded, and cut into 1-inch cubes
- 4 cups chicken stock
- ½ cube chicken bouillon
- One pinch of ground cumin
- One pinch ground allspice
- salt and ground black pepper to taste

Directions:
- ➢ Melt the butter in a large saucepan over medium heat; sauté the onion, garlic, and thyme in the hot butter for 5 minutes, or until the onion has softened. Bring the squash and chicken stock to a boil and cook for 10 to 15 minutes, or until the squash is soft. Pour in the bouillon, season with cumin, allspice, salt, and pepper, and remove from heat.
- ➢ Fill the blender no more than halfway with the soup. Hold the blender's lid in place with a kitchen towel and carefully start the blender, using a few fast pulses to get the soup flowing before leaving it on to puree. Puree in batches until smooth, then transfer to a serving basin. Alternatively, you may purée the soup in the pot using a stick blender.

Quick Creamy Zucchini Soup
Preparation Time: 10 minutes
Cooking Time: 15 minutes
Servings: 1

Ingredients:
- 4 cups shredded zucchini
- ¾ cup water
- ¾ teaspoon salt
- ½ teaspoon basil
- 2 cups warm milk
- Three tablespoons of all-purpose flour
- ½ teaspoon salt
- Three tablespoons butter
- Two tablespoons of minced onion
- ground black pepper to taste

Directions:
- ➢ In a saucepan, combine zucchini, water, salt, and basil; bring to a boil, decrease the heat to medium-low, and cook until zucchini is soft, about 15 minutes.
- ➢ Fill a blender halfway with the zucchini mixture. Cover and hold the lid down; pulse a few times before blending until smooth. Puree in small batches.
- ➢ In a mixing basin, combine warm milk, flour, and salt until smooth.
- ➢ In a pan over medium heat, melt the butter. 5 to 7 minutes, cook and toss the onion in heated butter until transparent. Pour in the pureed zucchini and milk mixture; bring to a boil, constantly stirring—season with pepper to taste.

The World's Best Tortilla Soup
Preparation Time: 10 minutes
Cooking Time: 15 minutes
Servings: 1

Ingredients:
- One tablespoon of vegetable oil
- One white onion, diced
- Two cloves of garlic, diced
- 1 (32 ounces) can of chicken broth
- 1 (14.5 ounces) can of chicken broth
- 1 (15 ounces) can of diced tomatoes
- Four large fresh tomatoes, diced
- 2 Anaheim chile peppers, stemmed and seeded

- One jalapeno pepper stemmed and seeded (Optional)
- Two tablespoons of ground cumin
- Two teaspoons of chilli powder
- One teaspoon of ground black pepper
- One whole rotisserie chicken, torn into bite-sized pieces
- One lime, sliced into wedges
- 3 cups crushed corn chips
- 1 (8 ounces) container of sour cream
- 1 (8 ounces) package of shredded Cheddar cheese
- One avocado - peeled, seeded, and sliced
- Three sprigs of cilantro, diced

Directions:
- In a large stockpot over medium heat, heat the vegetable oil. Cook and stir for 5 minutes, or until the onion and garlic are golden and soft. Mix in 2 cans of chicken broth and two cans of canned tomatoes. Toss in some fresh tomatoes.
- Combine Anaheim chile peppers, jalapeno peppers, cumin, chilli powder, and pepper in the saucepan. Incorporate the chicken. Bring to a boil; decrease the heat to medium and simmer the soup for 20 minutes, or until flavours merge.
- Pour soup into serving dishes and top with one lime wedge: corn chips, sour cream, Cheddar cheese, avocado slices, and cilantro.

Chilled Zucchini Soup

Preparation Time: 10 minutes
Cooking Time: 15 minutes

Servings: 1

Ingredients:
- Three tablespoons of olive oil, divided
- One onion, finely chopped
- Four fresh tomatoes, seeded and chopped
- 4 cups water
- Six sprigs of fresh mint, divided
- Three zucchini, sliced
- One tablespoon cornstarch
- One tablespoon of cold water
- salt and pepper to taste
- One teaspoon lemon juice, or to taste
- Two sprigs of fresh basil

Directions:
- In a large saucepan over medium heat, heat two tablespoons of olive oil and saute onion until tender and transparent, about 5 minutes. Cook for 2 minutes, stirring regularly, after adding the tomatoes.
- Bring the water to a boil in a saucepan. 4 sprigs of mint and four sprigs of zucchini. Reduce the heat to low and cover the soup for 15 minutes. Remove the mint.
- Combine cornstarch and cold water and add to soup. Increase the heat to medium and whisk in the cornstarch mixture until the soup thickens—season with salt and pepper to taste. Remove from the heat and leave to cool.
- Refrigerate soup for 2 hours or until it is cold. Before serving, drizzle with lemon juice and garnish with leftover mint, basil, and olive oil.

CHAPTER 12: SANDWICHES

Baked Eggplant Sandwiches

Preparation Time: 10 minutes
Cooking Time: 15 minutes
Servings: 1

Ingredients:

- Two tablespoons of olive oil, divided
- 2 cups panko bread crumbs
- Two teaspoons salt
- ½ teaspoon ground black pepper
- 1 cup all-purpose flour
- One egg
- ¼ cup water
- One large long eggplant, cut crosswise into 1/3 inch thick slices
- ½ cup finely chopped onion
- Three cloves of garlic, minced
- 5 ounces of fresh goat cheese
- 1 cup shredded sharp provolone cheese
- Two tablespoons of chopped fresh parsley
- Two tablespoons of chopped fresh basil leaves
- ground black pepper to taste
- ½ cup pomegranate molasses

Directions:

- ➤ Preheat the oven carefully to 450 degrees Fahrenheit (230 degrees C). Brush olive oil onto two large baking sheets.
- ➤ Combine the panko crumbs, salt, and 1/2 teaspoon of pepper in a medium mixing bowl. Whisk together the egg and water in a separate bowl. In a third bowl, combine the flour and baking powder. Coat each eggplant slice in flour, brushing off the excess, then in egg, and finally in panko crumbs. Place them on greased baking pans.
- ➤ Bake for 12 minutes in a preheated oven, flip the slices over and bake for another 12 minutes, or until golden brown. Remove from the oven and set aside to cool somewhat, but keep the oven on.
- ➤ Heat one tablespoon of oil in a pan over medium heat while the eggplant bakes. Cook and stir until the onion is almost soft, then add the garlic. Cook for approximately 1 minute. Take the pan off the heat and add the goat cheese, provolone cheese, parsley, and basil—season with pepper to taste.
- ➤ Divide the cheese mixture among eight eggplant pieces (half)—cover with remaining eggplant slices, pressing down to compress. Return the baking sheets to the oven.
- ➤ Bake for about 15 minutes or until the eggplant is crisp. Drizzle pomegranate molasses over two sandwiches on each serving platter.

Curried Egg Sandwiches

Preparation Time: 10 minutes
Cooking Time: 15 minutes
Servings: 1

Ingredients:

- Four hard-cooked eggs, peeled and chopped
- ½ cup mayonnaise
- One teaspoon of curry powder
- salt and pepper to taste
- Eight slices bread

Directions:

- ➤ In a mixing dish, combine mayonnaise and curry powder. Gently fold the eggs, then season with salt and pepper to taste. Divide evenly between 4 slices of bread, then top with the remaining four slices.

Chicken Salad Tea Sandwiches

Preparation Time: 10 minutes
Cooking Time: 15 minutes
Servings: 1

Ingredients:

- 1 (12.5 fl oz) can of white chunked chicken breast, drained
- One large Granny Smith apple - peeled, cored, and cut into small pieces
- ⅓ cup walnut halves
- ⅓ cup mayonnaise
- ½ teaspoon dried basil
- ¼ teaspoon dried dill weed
- One pinch salt
- Ten slices of good-quality white bread, crusts removed

Directions:

- ➤ In a food processor, combine the chicken, apple, walnuts, mayonnaise, basil, dill, and salt and pulse until well combined.
- ➤ Spread the chicken mixture onto the bread and top with another piece to make a sandwich. Continue with the remaining slices and mixture. Serve the sandwiches in quarters.

Mozzarella Meatball Sandwiches

Preparation Time: 10 minutes
Cooking Time: 15 minutes
Servings: 1

Ingredients:

- 1 (11.75 ounces) loaf Pepperidge Farm® Frozen Mozzarella Garlic Cheese Bread
- ½ cup Prego® Traditional Italian Sauce or Prego® Organic Tomato & Basil Italian Sauce
- 6 (1 ounce) frozen meatballs

Directions:

- ➤ Preheat the oven carefully to 400°F.
- ➤ Take the bread out of the bag. Place the frozen bread halves on an ungreased baking sheet, cut-side up. (If the bread halves are frozen together, delicately separate them with a fork.) Place a baking sheet in the centre of the oven.
- ➤ Bake for 10 minutes or until the mixture is heated.
- ➤ In a 2-quart saucepan, simmer the sauce and meatballs over low heat. Cook and stir for 20 minutes, or until the meatballs are well cooked.
- ➤ Place the meatballs on the bottom half of the bread. Top with the other half of the bread. Divide into quarters.

Salmon and Chive Tea Sandwiches

Preparation Time: 10 minutes
Cooking Time: 15 minutes
Servings: 1

Ingredients:

- 1 (8 ounces) container chive cream cheese
- 1 (1 pound) loaf of dark rye bread, thinly sliced
- ½ pound smoked salmon

Directions:

- ➤ On two pieces of bread, spread a thin layer of cream cheese. One slice sandwich with a tiny quantity of smoked salmon crumbled on top Seal the package and gently cut off the crust. Divide the crustless sandwich in half. Continue with the remaining ingredients.

Oven SPAM® Sandwiches

Preparation Time: 10 minutes
Cooking Time: 15 minutes
Servings: 1

Ingredients:
- 1 (12 ounces) can fully cook luncheon meat (such as SPAM®), cubed
- ¾ (1 pound) loaf of processed cheese food (such as Velveeta®), cubed
- Two tablespoons of sweet pickle relish
- ½ cup creamy salad dressing (such as Miracle Whip®)
- Eight hamburger buns, split

Directions:
- Preheat the oven carefully to 350°F (175 degrees C).
- Combine the luncheon meat, processed cheese, relish, and salad dressing in a mixing dish. Fill the sandwich buns with the filling, then wrap each sandwich individually in aluminium foil. Position the sandwiches on a baking sheet.
- Bake for 10 to 15 minutes, or until the hot filling and the buns are toasted.

Healthier Breakfast Sandwiches

Preparation Time: 10 minutes
Cooking Time: 15 minutes
Servings: 1

Ingredients:
- 2 pounds pork sausage
- One zucchini, finely chopped
- One pinch of red pepper flakes, or to taste
- ½ (8 ounces) package of fat-free cream cheese, or as needed
- Ten whole wheat English muffins, split
- 1 cup fresh spinach, or to taste

Directions:
- Combine the sausage, zucchini, and red pepper flakes in a mixing dish. Form the ingredients into ten patties.
- In a pan over medium heat, cook patties until no longer pink in the middle, 5 to 7 minutes per side. In the middle, an instant-read thermometer should read at least 160 degrees F. (70 degrees C).
- Spread cream cheese on English muffins and top with cooked burgers and spinach.

Ham Pineapple Sandwiches

Preparation Time: 10 minutes
Cooking Time: 15 minutes
Servings: 1

Ingredients:
- 1 (15 ounces) can of crushed pineapple, drained
- 1 cup white sugar
- 1 cup chopped walnuts
- 1 package of cream cheese
- Two tablespoons milk
- 24 slices of whole-grain bread
- 60 thin slices of deli ham

Directions:
- Combine the pineapple and sugar in a saucepan. Bring to a boil, then simmer, frequently stirring, for 5 to 10 minutes, or until thickened. Remove from the heat and set aside to cool. When the mixture has cooled, whisk in the walnuts.
- Soften the cream cheese in a medium mixing bowl, then add enough milk to make it spreadable. Incorporate the pineapple mixture. This component can be prepared the day before if desired.
- Two teaspoons of pineapple mixture are spread on one side of 12 pieces of bread, with five thin slices of ham on each. Finish with the remaining bread slices.

Funeral Sandwiches

Preparation Time: 10 minutes
Cooking Time: 15 minutes
Servings: 1

Ingredients:
- cooking spray
- 1 pound thinly sliced ham
- ½ pound sliced Swiss cheese
- 2 (12 counts) packages of Hawaiian bread rolls (such as King's®)
- 1 cup butter, melted
- Four tablespoons of brown sugar
- Two tablespoons of Worcestershire sauce
- Two tablespoons of prepared yellow mustard
- Two tablespoons of poppy seeds

Directions:
- Coat a baking sheet with cooking spray. Cover the bottoms of the buns with ham and Swiss cheese slices.
- Spread over sandwich tops, and combine the butter, brown sugar, Worcestershire sauce, mustard, and poppy seeds. Allow sitting for 4 hours to overnight.
- Preheat the oven carefully to 400° F. (200 degrees C).
- Bake for about 25 minutes, or until brown and the cheese has melted.

Barbeque Sauce for Meat Sandwiches

Preparation Time: 10 minutes
Cooking Time: 15 minutes
Servings: 1

Ingredients:
- 1 cup ketchup
- Two tablespoons of brown sugar
- Two tablespoons of Worcestershire sauce
- Two tablespoons honey
- One tablespoon butter
- One tablespoon of prepared mustard
- One tablespoon of lemon juice
- 1 ½ teaspoon chilli powder
- ¼ teaspoon garlic powder

Directions:
- In a saucepan over medium heat, combine ketchup, brown sugar, Worcestershire sauce, honey, butter, mustard, lemon juice, chilli powder, and garlic powder; cook until about 5 minutes.

Grilled Cheese and Tomato Sandwiches

Preparation Time: 10 minutes
Cooking Time: 15 minutes
Servings: 1

Ingredients:
- Four slices of whole-grain bread
- One tablespoon Country Crock® Spread
- One medium tomato, sliced
- 4 ounces sliced Cheddar cheese

Directions:
- Over medium heat, heat a 12-inch nonstick skillet. Distribute Country Crock® Spread on one side of each slice of bread.
- In a pan, place two slices, spread side down. Top each with a tomato, then a piece of cheese, and finally the last bread slice, spread side up.
- Cook until one side is lightly browned. Cook until the cheese is melted on the other side.

Sassy Tailgate Sandwiches

Preparation Time: 10 minutes
Cooking Time: 15 minutes
Servings: 1

Ingredients:

- 1 (12 counts) package of Hawaiian bread rolls
- 1 pound shaved Black Forest ham
- 12 slices Gruyere cheese
- 1 (8 ounces) tub PHILADELPHIA Chive & Onion Cream Cheese Spread
- ½ cup butter, melted
- One tablespoon of Worcestershire sauce
- ½ tablespoon dried minced onion
- ¼ cup grated Parmesan cheese

Directions:
- ➢ All rolls should be cut in half. Place the bottoms of the rolls in a 9x13-inch baking pan.
- ➢ Place an equal amount of ham on the bottom of each bun. Garnish with Gruyere.
- ➢ Spread a liberal quantity of cream cheese spread on each roll top. Making sandwiches, return the tops to the bottoms.
- ➢ Combine the butter, Worcestershire sauce, onion, and Parmesan cheese separately. Allow at least 20 minutes for the sauce to soak into the sandwiches. (You can prepare these ahead of time and store them in the refrigerator overnight.)
- ➢ Place the sandwiches, foil-wrapped, in a preheated 350°F oven—Bake for 20 minutes, or until well warmed. Enjoy!

Shredded Chicken Sandwiches

Preparation Time: 10 minutes
Cooking Time: 15 minutes
Servings: 1

Ingredients:
- ¼ cup slivered almonds
- Two slices of white bread
- Two tablespoons of olive oil
- salt and ground black pepper to taste
- 3 (5 ounces) skinless, boneless chicken breast halves
- 6 cups chicken broth, or as needed
- Two tablespoons of salted butter
- Four large rolls or buns (3-1/2" dia)s brioche buns, halved

Directions:
- ➢ Preheat the oven carefully to 375° F. (190 degrees C).
- ➢ In a food processor, grind almonds into tiny crumbs. Pulse the bread, oil, salt, and pepper into coarse crumbs. Spread the mixture evenly on a rimmed baking sheet.
- ➢ Bake for 10 minutes, stirring halfway through, in a preheated oven. Place aside to cool.
- ➢ Season the chicken with salt and pepper, then set it in a single layer in a Dutch oven or deep pan and fill with chicken broth. Bring to a boil over medium heat, scraping the foam from the top. Reduce the heat to low, cover, and cook for 10 to 14 minutes, or until the chicken is no longer pink in the middle. In the middle, an instant-read thermometer should read at least 165 degrees F. (74 degrees C). Allow the chicken to cool slightly on a chopping board before shredding with two forks.
- ➢ Remove the sediments from the chicken broth.
- ➢ Return the chicken to the saucepan, followed by the bread crumb mixture and 4 cups of chicken broth. Cook, occasionally stirring, over medium heat until the mixture reduces and achieves the desired consistency, about 20 minutes. Season with salt and pepper to taste.
- ➢ In a pan over medium-low heat, melt the butter. Then, for 1 to 2 minutes, toast the flat sides of the buns until golden brown. Serve with a large scoop of chicken mixture.

Hot Shredded Chicken Sandwiches

Preparation Time: 10 minutes
Cooking Time: 15 minutes
Servings: 1

Ingredients:
- 1 (3 pounds) chicken - cooked, deboned and shredded

- 2 (10.75 ounces) cans of condensed cream of mushroom soup
- ½ teaspoon poultry seasoning
- ¼ (16 ounces) package of buttery round crackers, crushed
- 12 hamburger buns

Directions:
- ➢ Combine the shredded chicken, condensed soup, poultry seasoning, and crumbled crackers in a large saucepan over medium heat. Cook, stirring regularly, for 15 to 20 minutes, or until the mixture is hot. Serve with buns.

Grilled Peanut Butter Apple Sandwiches

Preparation Time: 10 minutes
Cooking Time: 15 minutes
Servings: 1

Ingredients:
- 1 Gala apple, peeled, cored, and thinly sliced
- ½ teaspoon white sugar
- ½ teaspoon ground cinnamon
- Eight tablespoons of creamy peanut butter
- Eight slices of whole wheat bread
- ¼ cup unsalted butter

Directions:
- ➢ In a small bowl, combine cinnamon and sugar. One tablespoon of peanut butter spread on one side of 8 slices of bread
- ➢ Arrange four pieces of bread with apple slices on top. Evenly distribute the cinnamon/sugar mixture over the apples. Place the remaining four pieces of bread, peanut butter side down, on top.
- ➢ In a large pan over medium heat, melt the butter. Fry sandwiches till golden brown, about 1 to 2 minutes per side.

Vegan Tofu Scramble Breakfast Sandwiches

Preparation Time: 10 minutes
Cooking Time: 15 minutes
Servings: 1

Ingredients:
- Two tablespoons of vegetable oil
- 1 (12 ounces) package of firm tofu, drained
- ¾ cup canned fire-roasted tomatoes, drained
- One medium red bell pepper, diced
- ½ medium yellow onion, diced
- Two cloves of garlic, minced
- 1 ½ tablespoon nutritional yeast
- 1 ½ tablespoons soy sauce
- ½ teaspoon red pepper flakes
- ½ teaspoon paprika
- ¼ teaspoon ground turmeric
- One pinch of salt to taste
- One tablespoon vegan mayonnaise, or to taste
- Five each sandwich buns, split
- 1 cup fresh spinach
- One avocado, sliced

Directions:
- ➢ In a large skillet over medium heat, heat the oil. Crumble the tofu into 1-inch pieces and add to the pan. Cook for 5 minutes, stirring periodically. Cook until the extra liquid from the canned tomatoes has evaporated, 5 to 10 minutes. Cook until the bell pepper and onion is transparent, about 5 minutes. Combine the garlic, nutritional yeast, soy sauce, red pepper flakes, paprika, turmeric, and salt in a mixing bowl. Cook and stir for another 2 minutes.
- ➢ Top sandwich buns with mayonnaise, tofu mixture, spinach, and avocado.

Make-Ahead Turkey Tea Sandwiches

Preparation Time: 10 minutes
Cooking Time: 15 minutes
Servings: 1

Ingredients:
- ½ cup low-fat cream cheese softened
- One teaspoon of minced garlic
- ½ teaspoon Italian seasoning
- 1 French baguette
- 4 ounces thinly sliced cooked deli turkey
- 1 cup baby spinach leaves, or to taste
- ½ red bell pepper, thinly sliced
- ½ cup artichoke hearts, drained and chopped
- toothpicks

Directions:
- ➢ Set aside the cream cheese, garlic, and Italian seasoning in a small bowl.
- ➢ Using a serrated knife, cut the top third of the baguette off. Remove a 1/2-inch shell by scooping off a portion of the bottom half. Distribute the cream cheese mixture evenly between the two sides. Layer the bottom shell with turkey, spinach, red pepper, and artichokes, then top with the second half. Wrap securely in foil and place in the refrigerator for 2 hours or overnight.
- ➢ Uncover the loaf and cut it into 1- to 2-inch slices diagonally when ready to serve. Each is held together with a toothpick.

Slow Cooker Buffalo Chicken Sandwiches

Preparation Time: 10 minutes
Cooking Time: 15 minutes
Servings: 1

Ingredients:
- Four skinless, boneless chicken breast halves
- 1 (17.5 fluid ounce) bottle Buffalo wing sauce, divided
- ½ (1 ounce) package dry ranch salad dressing mix
- Two tablespoons butter
- Six hoagie rolls split lengthwise

Directions:
- ➢ Pour 3/4 of the wing sauce and ranch dressing combination over the chicken breasts in the slow cooker.
- ➢ Cook on Low for 6 to 7 hours, covered.
- ➢ With two forks, shred the chicken in the slow cooker. Stir in the butter.
- ➢ Pile the shredded chicken and sauce on top of the hoagie bread. Serve with any leftover Buffalo sauce.

Grilled Fish Sandwiches for Two

Preparation Time: 10 minutes
Cooking Time: 15 minutes
Servings: 1

Ingredients:
- One tablespoon of unsalted butter
- ½ teaspoon Creole seasoning
- 2 (6 ounces) fillets cod fillets
- ½ teaspoon smoked paprika
- Two tablespoons of vegetable oil
- Two each sub-style sandwich rolls, split
- Six leaves of romaine lettuce
- Four slices tomato
- Two tablespoons of remoulade sauce, or to taste

Directions:
- ➢ Preheat an outdoor grill to 375°F and clean the grates (190 degrees C).
- ➢ Melt butter and add Creole seasoning and smoked paprika to taste.
- ➢ Brush each side of the fillets with the seasoned butter mixture after drying them with a paper towel.
- ➢ Grill the fillets for 1 minute after carefully oiling the grill grates. Grill for 1 minute longer after gently rotating the fish on the grate 60 to 90 degrees to generate grill marks. Turn the fillets over using a fish turner and cook for 1 minute—grill for 1-minute longer after rotating. When the fish flakes easily with a fork and an instant-read thermometer placed into the middle reads 145 degrees F, it is done (63 degrees C).
- ➢ Place Romaine leaves and cooked fish into sandwich rolls. Serve with tomato slices on top. Serve with remoulade sauce.

Frozen Chocolate Graham's Ice Cream Sandwiches

Preparation Time: 10 minutes
Cooking Time: 15 minutes
Servings: 1

Ingredients:
- 20 whole chocolate graham crackers
- 1 container of frozen whipped topping

Directions:
- ➢ Chocolate graham crackers, cut into squares. Spread a heavy layer of whipped topping on half of the squares and sandwich with another square. Wrap in plastic wrap and place in the freezer for 1 hour or until firm.

CHAPTER 13: SEAFOOD

Mixed Seafood Curry

Preparation Time: 10 minutes
Cooking Time: 15 minutes
Servings: 1

Ingredients:
- Two tablespoons of vegetable oil
- One medium onion, halved and sliced
- One tablespoon minced fresh ginger root
- One tablespoon of minced garlic
- 1 can of light coconut milk
- Three tablespoons of lime juice
- One tablespoon curry paste, or more to taste
- One tablespoon of brown sugar
- 12 medium shrimp
- 12 sea scallops, halved
- 6 ounces asparagus
- Two tablespoons of chopped cilantro
- salt to taste

Directions:
- ➤ In a large skillet over medium-high heat, heat the oil. Cook onion, ginger, and garlic in heated oil for 2 to 3 minutes, or until the onion begins to soften. Stir in the coconut milk, lime juice, curry paste, and brown sugar, then bring to a boil and cook for 5 minutes, or until slightly reduced.
- ➤ Cook until the shrimp and scallops are no longer clear in the middle, approximately 5 minutes. Stir in the asparagus, cilantro, and salt.

Sophia's Homemade Seafood Stock

Preparation Time: 10 minutes
Cooking Time: 15 minutes
Servings: 1

Ingredients:
- One tablespoon of olive oil
- Two large onions, coarsely chopped
- One bunch of celery, coarsely chopped
- Four large carrots, coarsely chopped
- Two large green bell peppers, coarsely chopped
- One bunch of fresh cilantro
- ½ bunch of fresh oregano
- Two bay leaves
- 3 ½ (1 litre) bottles of water
- ½ pound fish parts (such as bones, spine, and tail)
- Two large fish heads
- 2 cups clam juice
- One teaspoon of whole black peppercorns

Directions:
- ➤ In a large stockpot, heat the olive oil over medium-high heat. For 5 minutes, cook and sauté onions in heated oil. Cook for 5 minutes more after adding the celery, carrots, and bell peppers. Combine the cilantro, oregano, and bay leaves in a mixing bowl. Cook for another 2 minutes. Combine the water, fish pieces, fish heads, clam juice, and peppercorns in a mixing bowl.
- ➤ Bring the mixture to a boil, lower to low heat, and leave uncovered for at least 4 hours. Please turn off the heat and set it aside for 30 minutes to cool.
- ➤ Using a skimmer or slotted spoon, remove bulk things from the stock. Strain stock into a large container using a fine-mesh strainer, ensuring all fish bones are removed. Use immediately or freeze for later.

Seafood Sausage

Preparation Time: 10 minutes
Cooking Time: 15 minutes
Servings: 1

Ingredients:
- Two tablespoons of butter, or to taste, divided
- Two tablespoons of minced shallot
- 8 ounces boneless, skinless sole, chilled and cubed
- 1 (4 ounces) skinless salmon fillet, chilled and cubed
- 4 ounces shrimp - chilled, peeled, deveined, and chopped
- Two tablespoons of plain dry breadcrumbs
- Four large egg whites
- One large egg
- Two teaspoons of kosher salt
- Two pinches of cayenne pepper, or to taste
- Two tablespoons of chopped Italian parsley
- For the Sauce:
- Two tablespoons water
- One lemon, juiced
- Two tablespoons of cold butter
- One tablespoon of chopped Italian parsley
- salt to taste

Directions:
- ➤ In a pan over medium-high heat, melt two teaspoons of butter. Saute shallots for 5 minutes or until softened and sweetened. Allow cooling till room temperature.
- ➤ In a food processor, combine the sole, salmon, and shrimp. Mix in the bread crumbs. Add the egg whites and entire egg—season with cayenne pepper and kosher salt. Combine the shallots and parsley when they have cooled.
- ➤ Cover the processor and pulse on and off, beginning with brief pulses and progressing to longer pulses, until the mixture is well mixed and clumps together at the blade. Wrap the mixture in plastic wrap and place it in the refrigerator for 1 to 2 hours.
- ➤ 1/4 of the sausage mixture should be placed on a piece of plastic wrap. Form into a log using moistened fingertips. Wrap the plastic around the roll, twisting the ends to seal. Roll up the log onto a piece of aluminium foil. Twist the ends together, but not too firmly. Fold the ends in. Repeat with the rest of the sausage mixture.
- ➤ Bring a saucepan of water to a gentle boil. Add the sausages and cover with a plate. Simmer on low for 20 minutes, covered.
- ➤ To halt the cooking process, place the sausages in a dish of cold water. Allow 15 to 20 minutes to cool. Remove from the water and place in the refrigerator until ready to serve.
- ➤ Remove the foil off the sausages with a paper towel. Snip one end of the plastic wrap and squeeze the sausage through it. Remove any unappealing bits.
- ➤ Melt the remaining butter in a small saucepan over medium heat. Cook the sausages in the heated butter, often rotating, for 5 to 6 minutes, or until browned all over. Cover and reduce the heat to medium-low. Cook for 5 to 6 minutes more, or until an instant-read thermometer inserted into the sausages registers 140 degrees F (60 degrees C). Rep with the remaining sausages.
- ➤ Bring water and lemon juice to a boil in the same pan. Cook until the liquid has been reduced by half, about 3 minutes. Reduce the heat to low and stir in the parsley and cooled butter. Swirl the pan until butter is melted, then season with salt and swirl again. Pour the sauce over the sausages.

Seafood Lasagna II

Preparation Time: 10 minutes
Cooking Time: 15 minutes
Servings: 1

Ingredients:

- 1 (16 ounces) package of lasagna noodles
- Two tablespoons of olive oil
- One clove of garlic, minced
- 1 pound baby portobello mushrooms, sliced
- 2 (16 ounces) jars of Alfredo-style pasta sauce
- 1 pound shrimp, peeled and deveined
- 1 pound bay scallops
- 1 pound imitation crabmeat, chopped
- 20 ounces ricotta cheese
- One egg
- black pepper
- 6 cups shredded Italian cheese blend

Directions:

- ➢ Preheat the oven carefully to 350°F (175 degrees C). Warm up a big saucepan of gently salted water. Cook for 8 to 10 minutes, or until pasta is al dente; drain.
- ➢ In a large saucepan over medium heat, heat the oil. Cook until the garlic and mushrooms are soft. Add two jars of Alfredo sauce. Add the shrimp, scallops, and crabmeat and mix well. Simmer for 5 to 10 minutes, or until well cooked. Combine the ricotta cheese, egg, and pepper in a medium mixing basin.
- ➢ Layer noodles, ricotta mixture, Alfredo mixture, and shredded cheese in a 9x13 baking dish. Layer until all ingredients are utilized, ensuring shredded cheese on top.
- ➢ Bake for 45 minutes, uncovered, in a preheated oven. Bake for 15 minutes, covered.

Seafood Mocequa

Preparation Time: 10 minutes
Cooking Time: 15 minutes
Servings: 1

Ingredients:

- 2 pounds firm white fish, such as monkfish, cut into 2-inch pieces
- ½ pound medium shrimp, peeled and deveined
- salt and pepper to taste
- Three tablespoons of dende oil (red palm oil) or canola
- One onion, cut into 1/2-inch pieces
- One tablespoon of minced garlic
- Two tomatoes, seeded and diced
- One red bell pepper, chopped
- of 2 long, hot peppers, seeded and chopped
- ½ cup fish stock
- ¼ cup chopped fresh cilantro
- One bunch of green onions, diced
- Two bay leaves
- 1 ½ teaspoon hot pepper sauce (e.g. Tabasco™), or to taste
- ½ cup coconut milk

Directions:

- ➢ Set aside. Toss the fish and shrimp with salt and pepper to taste. In a large skillet over medium heat, heat the dende oil. Cook until the onions are softened and transparent. Cook until the onions are golden brown, then add the garlic.
- ➢ Heat for 5 minutes after adding the tomato, add the red and spicy peppers and cook until softened. Combine the fish stock, cilantro, green onions, bay leaves, and spicy sauce in a mixing bowl. Bring to a boil over medium-high heat, lower to medium and continue to cook until reduced by 1/4.
- ➢ Pour in the coconut milk, followed by the fish. Simmer the fish until it is firm and opaque. Serve right away.

Eric and Debi's Seafood Ceviche

Preparation Time: 10 minutes

Cooking Time: 15 minutes
Servings: 1

Ingredients:

- ½ pound halibut fillets, cut into 1/4 inch cubes
- Ten peeled and deveined shrimp, cut into small pieces
- Four large sea scallops, cut into small pieces
- ½ cup fresh lemon juice
- ¼ cup fresh grapefruit juice
- One yellow bell pepper, diced
- Three large jalapeno peppers, seeded and minced
- ⅓ cup diced Maui onion
- ¼ cup chopped green olives
- One tablespoon minced fresh ginger root
- One tablespoon of brown sugar
- One teaspoon salt
- 1 (6 ounces) can of tomato paste
- One large tomato, diced

Directions:

- ➢ Combine the halibut, shrimp, scallops, lemon juice, and grapefruit juice in a glass bowl. Refrigerate for at least 6 hours or until the halibut becomes opaque.
- ➢ In a glass dish, combine the bell pepper, jalapeño pepper, onion, olives, ginger, sugar, salt, and tomato paste until no tomato paste lumps remain. Drain the fish and combine it with the vegetables and tomatoes. Return to the refrigerator to cool for at least 15 minutes before serving, stirring gently.

Spicy Tomato, Seafood, and Chorizo Stew

Preparation Time: 10 minutes
Cooking Time: 15 minutes
Servings: 1

Ingredients:

- One tablespoon of olive oil
- One onion, chopped
- Two each poblano peppers, seeded and chopped
- Three cloves of garlic, minced
- 8 ounces chorizo sausage
- 1 (32 ounces) container of chicken stock or broth
- 2 (14.5 ounce) cans Hunt's® no salt added Petite Diced Tomatoes, drained
- 1 (11 ounces) can of Mexican-style corn, drained
- 1 (7 ounces) can make salsa verde
- 1 ½ teaspoon ground cumin
- ½ teaspoon ground chipotle chile pepper, or to taste
- 1 pound cod fillets (or another firm white fish like halibut), cut into chunks
- 1 pound large raw shrimp, peeled, deveined
- 1 Chopped green onions
- One bunch of Chopped fresh cilantro
- 1 Lime wedges

Directions:

- ➢ In a large skillet over medium heat, heat the olive oil. Cook and stir until the onion, peppers, and garlic are tender, 5 to 7 minutes. Place on a platter. Cook, constantly stirring, until the ground chorizo is browned and cooked through 5 to 7 minutes. Turn off the heat.
- ➢ Fill a large soup pot halfway with chicken stock. Combine Hunt's tomatoes, Mexican corn, salsa verde, cumin, chipotle, and softened onion-pepper-garlic combination in a mixing bowl. Stir everything together, then simmer for 10 minutes to let the flavours merge.
- ➢ Continue to boil for 5 to 7 minutes, or until the cod, shrimp, and saved chorizo is cooked.
- ➢ Serve in serving dishes. Serve with chopped fresh green onions, cilantro, and lime wedges.

Savannah Seafood Stuffing

Preparation Time: 10 minutes

Cooking Time: 15 minutes
Servings: 1

Ingredients:

- ½ cup margarine
- ½ cup chopped green bell pepper
- ½ cup chopped onion
- ½ cup chopped celery
- 1 pound crabmeat, drained and flaked
- ½ pound medium shrimp - peeled and deveined
- ½ cup seasoned dry bread crumbs
- 1 (6 ounces) package of cornbread stuffing mix
- Two tablespoons of white sugar, divided
- 1 (10.75 ounces) can of condensed cream of mushroom soup
- 1 (14.5 ounces) can of chicken broth

Directions:

- ➢ In a large pan over medium heat, melt the margarine. Cook and stir for 5 minutes with the bell pepper, onion, celery, crabmeat, and shrimp. Place aside. In a large mixing basin, combine the filling, bread crumbs, and one tablespoon of sugar. Mix in the skillet veggies and fish. Mix in the cream of mushroom soup and as much chicken broth as desired. Pour into a 9x13 baking dish.
- ➢ Bake for 30 minutes, or until gently browned on top, in a preheated oven.

Kahala's Macaroni Seafood Salad

Preparation Time: 10 minutes
Cooking Time: 15 minutes
Servings: 1

Ingredients:

- 1 (16 ounces) package spaghetti, broken into 2-inch pieces
- Four hard-cooked eggs, chopped
- One carrot, grated
- ½ cup frozen petite peas, thawed
- 1 cup frozen fully cooked salad shrimp, thawed
- ½ cup crab meat, cooked
- 16 ounces mayonnaise
- ¼ cup milk
- One teaspoon of lemon juice
- One teaspoon sugar
- salt to taste
- black pepper to taste
- paprika to taste

Directions:

- ➢ Boil a big kettle of lightly salted water. Cook until the pasta is al dente, about 8 to 10 minutes. Drain the pasta and place it in a large mixing bowl. Incorporate the eggs, carrots, peas, shrimp, and crab meat. Refrigerate, covered.
- ➢ Combine mayonnaise, milk, lemon juice, and sugar in a mixing bowl to create the dressing—season with salt, pepper, and paprika to taste.
- ➢ Stir the dressing into the cooled spaghetti until fully blended. If the salad appears to be dry, add extra mayonnaise and a splash of milk or water before serving, cover and chill.

Seafood Chili

Preparation Time: 10 minutes
Cooking Time: 15 minutes
Servings: 1

Ingredients:

- ¼ cup butter
- Four fresh tomatoes, diced
- Two bell peppers, chopped into 3/4 inch pieces
- Two heads of garlic, crushed
- Three green onions, chopped
- 1 (8 ounces) can of kidney beans, drained

- 1 (8 ounces) can of baby corn, drained and cut into bite-size pieces
- Two stalks of celery, chopped
- One tablespoon chilli powder, or to taste
- One dash of lime juice, or to taste
- 1 (16 ounces) can of whole peeled tomatoes, with liquid
- ½ pound cooked crabmeat
- 1 pinch brown sugar, or as needed (Optional)
- 1 (7 ounces) can hearts of palm, drained and cut into bite-size pieces
- 1 pound jumbo shrimp - peeled, deveined, and tails removed
- 1 pound sea scallops
- sea salt and freshly ground black pepper to taste

Directions:

- ➢ In a large stockpot over medium-low heat, melt the butter; add the tomatoes, bell peppers, garlic, and green onions. Cook, stirring regularly, for 30 minutes to 1 hour, or until tomatoes are virtually liquefied.
- ➢ Stir in the kidney beans, baby corn, celery, chilli powder and lime juice, and season with salt and powdered black pepper. Cook, covered, over low heat for 1 hour, or until celery is tender but still has firmness.
- ➢ Stir in crab meat and canned tomatoes with juice, breaking up tomatoes in thirds with a wooden spoon. Season with salt and pepper; add brown sugar if the chilli is too salty.
- ➢ Cook until the shrimp, scallops, and hearts of palm are brilliant pink on the exterior and the flesh is opaque, 2 to 3 minutes.

Sunomono (Japanese Cucumber and Seafood Salad)

Preparation Time: 10 minutes
Cooking Time: 15 minutes
Servings: 1

Ingredients:

- One large English cucumber, peeled and thinly sliced
- One teaspoon salt
- 1 (8 ounces) package of imitation crab sticks, halved
- Two tablespoons of rice vinegar
- One tablespoon of soy sauce
- One teaspoon of sesame seeds, or to taste

Directions:

- ➢ Place cucumber slices on a large platter and season both sides with salt. Set aside for about 15 minutes, or until the cucumber has lost its water. Brush the salt off the cucumbers and flatten them with a paper towel to remove any extra moisture.
- ➢ In a glass dish bowl, combine cucumber slices, crab sticks, rice vinegar, and soy sauce; toss to coat. Refrigerate for at least 1 hour after wrapping the bowl in plastic wrap (or 24 hours).
- ➢ Divide the cucumber salad among four dishes and top with sesame seeds.

Easy Seafood Alfredo

Preparation Time: 10 minutes
Cooking Time: 15 minutes
Servings: 1

Ingredients:

- One tablespoon butter
- Three cloves of garlic, minced
- ½ cup chicken broth
- 1 cup fat-free half-and-half
- Six tablespoons of grated Parmesan cheese
- One slice of fat-free American cheese, torn into pieces
- One teaspoon of dried basil
- One teaspoon of dried parsley
- ground black pepper to taste

- 2 (8 ounces) packages of imitation crabmeat, flaked

Directions:
- ➢ Warm up a big saucepan of gently salted water. Cook for 8 to 10 minutes, or until pasta is al dente, then drain.
- ➢ In a pan over medium heat, melt the butter and sauté the garlic for 1 minute. Pour in the half-and-half and chicken broth. Cook and stir until well cooked.
- ➢ In the pan, combine the Parmesan and American cheeses. Cook, constantly stirring, until the American cheese melts. Season with basil, parsley, and pepper to taste. Continue frying until the imitation crabmeat is cooked completely. Serve with cooked spaghetti.

Paleo Seafood Chili

Preparation Time: 10 minutes
Cooking Time: 15 minutes
Servings: 1

Ingredients:
- One tablespoon of olive oil
- One large onion, chopped
- One red bell pepper, chopped
- One green bell pepper, chopped
- Two stalks of celery, chopped
- Three cloves of garlic, minced
- 1 ½ teaspoons sea salt, divided
- One teaspoon freshly ground pepper, divided
- 1 (15 ounces) can of diced tomatoes
- 1 cup chicken broth
- One tablespoon of dried parsley
- Two teaspoons of chilli powder
- ¾ teaspoon cayenne pepper
- One tablespoon of tomato paste
- ½ pound sea scallops - rinsed, drained, patted dry, and cut in half
- ½ pound haddock, cut into cubes
- ½ pound uncooked medium shrimp, peeled and deveined

Directions:
- ➢ In a big heavy saucepan, heat the olive oil over medium-high heat. Cook until the onion, red bell pepper, green bell pepper, celery, and garlic are softened, 3 to 4 minutes. Add 1/2 teaspoon salt and 1/2 teaspoon pepper to taste. Bring the tomatoes and broth to a boil. Turn the heat down to medium-low. Cook until thickened, approximately 15 minutes, with the parsley, chilli powder, and cayenne pepper. Stir in the tomato paste until it has dissolved.
- ➢ Season the scallops and haddock with the remaining one teaspoon salt and 1/2 teaspoon pepper and place in the pot. Cook until the shrimp are brilliant pink on the outside and opaque in the centre, about 7 minutes.

Layered Seafood Dip

Preparation Time: 10 minutes
Cooking Time: 15 minutes
Servings: 1

Ingredients:
- 1 package of cream cheese
- ½ cup sour cream
- ¼ cup mayonnaise
- 1 cup cocktail sauce
- ½ cup chopped green bell pepper
- Three green onions, chopped
- One tomato, seeded and chopped
- 1 cup cooked crabmeat
- 1 cup cooked baby shrimp
- 1 cup finely shredded mozzarella cheese

Directions:
- ➢ Combine the cream cheese, sour cream, and mayonnaise in a medium mixing dish.

- ➢ Spread the cream cheese mixture on the bottom of a 12-inch circular serving dish. Pour the cocktail sauce over the mixture evenly. Layer green bell pepper, green onions, and tomato on top. Crabmeat and shrimp on top. Garnish with mozzarella.
- ➢ Refrigerate for at least 2 hours before serving, covered.

Spicy Seafood Shell Appetizers

Preparation Time: 10 minutes
Cooking Time: 15 minutes
Servings: 1

Ingredients:
- 1 ½ cups mayonnaise
- ⅔ cup grated Parmesan cheese
- ⅔ cup shredded Swiss cheese
- ⅓ cup chopped onion
- Two teaspoons of Worcestershire sauce
- Ten drops of hot pepper sauce
- 1 (4 ounces) can of small shrimp, drained
- 1 (6 ounces) can crabmeat, drained and flaked
- 2 (2.1 ounces) packages of mini phyllo tart shells
- paprika

Directions:
- ➢ Preheat the oven carefully to 400°F (200 degrees C). Grease a medium baking sheet lightly.
- ➢ In a medium mixing bowl, combine mayonnaise, Parmesan cheese, Swiss cheese, onion, Worcestershire sauce, and spicy pepper sauce. Stir in the shrimp and crabmeat gently.
- ➢ Make shells out of the phyllo dough. Fill shells halfway with the mixture.
- ➢ Place the filled shells on a baking sheet—Bake for 7 to 10 minutes, or until gently browned, in a preheated oven. Before serving, sprinkle with paprika.

Baked Seafood Au Gratin

Preparation Time: 10 minutes
Cooking Time: 15 minutes
Servings: 1

Ingredients:
- One onion, chopped
- One green bell pepper, chopped
- 1 cup butter, divided
- 1 cup all-purpose flour, divided
- 1 pound of fresh crabmeat
- 4 cups water
- 1 pound fresh shrimp, peeled and deveined
- ½ pound small scallops
- ½ pound flounder fillets
- 3 cups milk
- 1 cup shredded sharp Cheddar cheese
- One tablespoon of distilled white vinegar
- One teaspoon of Worcestershire sauce
- ½ teaspoon salt
- One pinch of ground black pepper
- One dash of hot pepper sauce
- ½ cup grated Parmesan cheese

Directions:
- ➢ Sauté the onion and pepper in 1/2 cup of butter in a large pan. Cook until vegetables are soft. Stir add 1/2 cup of the flour and simmer for 10 minutes over medium heat, stirring regularly. Remove from heat, stir in crabmeat, and put aside.
- ➢ Bring the water to a boil in a large Dutch oven. Simmer for 3 minutes after adding the shrimp, scallops, and flounder. Drain the seafood, reserving 1 cup of the cooking liquid, and put it aside.
- ➢ Melt the remaining 1/2 cup butter in a large saucepan over low heat. Add the remaining 1/2 cup flour and mix well. Cook for 1 minute, stirring regularly. Add the milk and 1 cup

of the leftover cooking liquid gradually. Raise the heat to be medium and cook, frequently stirring, until the sauce thickens and becomes bubbling. Combine the shredded Cheddar cheese, vinegar, Worcestershire sauce, salt, pepper, and spicy sauce in a large mixing bowl. Incorporate cooked fish.

➢ Preheat the oven carefully to 350°F (175 degrees C). Grease a 9x13-inch baking dish lightly. Fill the bottom of the prepared pan with the crabmeat mixture. Sprinkle the Parmesan cheese over the seafood combination and crabmeat crust.

➢ Bake for 30 minutes, or until gently browned, in a preheated oven. Serve right away.

Instant Pot® Seafood Chowder

Preparation Time: 10 minutes
Cooking Time: 15 minutes
Servings: 1

Ingredients:
- Four slices of bacon, cut into 1-inch pieces
- Five cloves of garlic, minced
- One medium onion, diced
- Three stalks of celery, thinly sliced
- One medium carrot, diced
- Four medium russet potatoes, peeled and cubed
- 1 (14 ounces) can of whole kernel corn
- 2 cups vegetable broth
- 6 (4 ounces) haddock fillets
- 1 cup uncooked medium shrimp
- 1 cup of sea scallops
- One tablespoon of chopped fresh thyme
- One pinch of red pepper flakes, or to taste
- ground black pepper to taste
- Two tablespoons cornstarch
- Two tablespoons water
- 1 cup milk

Directions:
➢ Select the Saute function on a multi-functional pressure cooker (such as an Instant Pot®). Brown the bacon for 5 to 7 minutes. Cook and stir for 30 seconds after adding the garlic. Add the onion, then the celery and carrot. Cook for 1 to 2 minutes, stirring constantly. Deactivate the Saute function.

➢ On top of the vegetable mixture, layer potatoes, then corn. Add the veggie broth. On top, layer haddock, shrimp, and scallops.

➢ Close the lid and secure it. Set the timer for 5 minutes and use high pressure as directed by the manufacturer. Allow 10 to 15 minutes for the pressure to rise.

➢ For 10 minutes, use the natural-release technique according to the manufacturer's recommendations. After about 5 minutes, carefully remove any leftover pressure using the quick-release technique as directed by the manufacturer. Remove the lid by unlocking it.

➢ Turn on the Saute function and swirl the fish to break it up. Thyme, red pepper flakes, and ground pepper are optional. In a measuring cup, combine cornstarch and water; add into the soup and boil until thickened. Pour in the milk and serve.

Sopa de Mariscos (Seafood Soup)

Preparation Time: 10 minutes
Cooking Time: 15 minutes
Servings: 1

Ingredients:
- Two tablespoons of olive oil
- One medium onion, chopped
- Two cloves of garlic, minced
- Three medium carrots, diced
- One ear of fresh corn, kernels cut from the cob
- One stalk of celery, halved and diced
- 6 cups chicken stock (such as Swanson®)
- 1 (10 ounces) can of diced tomatoes with green chile peppers
- 1 (10 ounces) can of diced tomatoes with green chile peppers, lime, and cilantro (such as RO*TEL®)
- One ancho chile pepper, diced
- One tablespoon of chilli powder
- Two teaspoons of ground cumin
- 1 pound fresh littleneck clams
- 1 pound of fresh mussels
- 1 pound fresh cod, cut into bite-sized pieces
- ¾ pound fresh shrimp, peeled and deveined
- ¼ cup fresh cilantro, chopped, or to taste
- One avocado, peeled and sliced

Directions:
➢ In a medium-sized stockpot, heat the olive oil. Cook until the onion is transparent, 5 to 7 minutes. Cook until the garlic is aromatic, approximately 1 minute.

➢ Cook until the carrots, corn, and celery are softened, about 5 minutes. Bring the chicken stock, tomatoes, ancho chilli, chilli powder, and cumin to a boil. Reduce the heat to low, cover, and leave to simmer for 45 minutes.

➢ Meanwhile, rinse the clams and mussels in cold water to remove any sand.

➢ Drain the clams and mussels and add them to the soup. Mix in the cod and shrimp. Cover and cook for 5 to 10 minutes, or until the fish is white and flaky, the mussels and clams are open, and the shrimp is pink. Serve immediately with cilantro and avocado on top.

Amazing Seafood Pasta with Lobster

Preparation Time: 10 minutes
Cooking Time: 15 minutes
Servings: 1

Ingredients:
- 1 (16 ounces) package bow-tie pasta
- Three tablespoons of butter, divided
- One tablespoon of finely diced shallot
- 2 cups heavy whipping cream
- ½ cup dry white wine (such as Chardonnay)
- cayenne pepper
- Two pinches saffron
- salt and ground black pepper to taste
- 1 pound uncooked shrimp - peeled, deveined, and tails removed
- ½ pound cooked lobster meat
- ½ pound cooked lump crabmeat
- lemon, juiced

Directions:
➢ Warm up a big saucepan of gently salted water. Boil bow-tie pasta for 12 minutes, tossing periodically, until soft yet firm to the bite. Drain, then whisk in 1 tablespoon of butter. Keep heated and set aside.

➢ In a large saucepan over medium heat, melt the remaining butter. Cook until the shallot is softened, about 1 minute. Bring the cream and wine to a boil: Cayenne pepper, saffron, salt, and black pepper to taste. Reduce the heat to a moderate simmer for 10 minutes to allow the sauce to thicken.

➢ Melt butter in a frying pan over medium heat. Cook until the shrimp are opaque, 3 to 5 minutes. Cook until the lobster and crab are cooked through, about 2 minutes longer. Season with salt and black pepper to taste.

➢ Stir the seafood mixture into the sauce in the saucepan. Simmer for 10 minutes more on low heat with the lemon juice.

➢ Serve cooked pasta in separate dishes, topped with two spoons of sauce. Gently fold the sauce into the spaghetti and season with black pepper to taste.

Psarosoupa (Greek Seafood Soup)

Preparation Time: 10 minutes
Cooking Time: 15 minutes
Servings: 1

Ingredients:

- 6 cups of seafood stock
- 2 pounds of swordfish steaks
- Four tablespoons of olive oil, divided or as needed
- ½ large white onion, diced
- Three medium carrots, sliced
- Three stalks of celery, sliced
- Four cloves of garlic, minced
- 1 (2 ounces) can of anchovies, minced
- Four tablespoons of lemon juice
- One tablespoon of fresh lemon zest
- Two tablespoons of chopped fresh parsley
- ½ tablespoon salt
- Two teaspoons of fresh celery leaves, chopped
- One teaspoon of ground black pepper
- One teaspoon of chopped fresh thyme
- One bay leaf
- Two medium russet potatoes, peeled and cubed
- ½ cup uncooked white rice
- salt and ground black pepper to taste

Directions:

➢ Bring the stock to a boil in a large stockpot. 5 to 6 minutes until swordfish is cooked through and readily flaked with a fork. Remove the fish from the stock, saving all of the liquid. Chop/tear the fish coarsely.

➢ Heat two tablespoons of olive oil in a separate saucepan over medium heat. Mix in the onion, carrots, and celery. After 5 minutes, add the garlic. One minute more sautéing. Pour in the saved stock. Combine anchovies, lemon juice and zest, parsley, 1/2 tablespoon salt, celery leaves, one teaspoon pepper, thyme, and bay leaf in a mixing bowl. Bring to a boil, then lower to medium-low heat. Allow flavours to mingle for around 20 minutes.

➢ Stir in the potatoes and rice and continue to cook until the rice and potatoes are cooked, about 20 minutes more, adding the swordfish in the final 5 minutes of cooking time. To taste, season with more salt and pepper.

➢ Pour soup into dishes and sprinkle with remaining olive oil.

CHAPTER 14: POULTRY

Indian Barbeque Chicken

Preparation Time: 10 minutes
Cooking Time: 15 minutes
Servings: 1

Ingredients:
- 3 pounds of bone-in chicken pieces
- Three tablespoons of fresh lemon juice
- One tablespoon meat tenderizer
- 2 cups plain yoghurt, divided
- Three tablespoons of ground cumin
- Two tablespoons of ground coriander
- ⅓ cup chopped fresh cilantro
- Two teaspoons paprika
- ½ teaspoon ground turmeric
- Two teaspoons salt
- One teaspoon of ground black pepper
- Six cloves of garlic, minced

Directions:
- ➢ To assist absorb more flavour, make small transverse incisions in the flesh of the chicken sections. Rub the lemon juice and meat tenderizer into the chicken flesh. Put the chicken in a shallow dish.
- ➢ In a blender or food processor, combine 1/2 cup yoghurt, cumin, coriander, cilantro, paprika, turmeric, salt, pepper, and garlic until smooth. Transfer to a mixing dish and toss in the remaining 1 1/2 cups of yoghurt. Cover and place the chicken pieces in the refrigerator for at least 8 hours or overnight.
- ➢ Preheat the grill to medium.
- ➢ Oil the grill grate lightly. Remove the chicken from the marinade and discard the marinade. Grill the chicken for 30 to 45 minutes, regularly rotating to avoid scorching, or until the juices flow clear. Smaller portions will be done initially.

Yellow Chicken

Preparation Time: 10 minutes
Cooking Time: 15 minutes
Servings: 1

Ingredients:
- Two tablespoons of olive oil
- One teaspoon of Worcestershire sauce
- One teaspoon of ground turmeric
- One teaspoon of dry mustard powder
- One clove of garlic, minced
- Four skinless, bone-in chicken breast halves
- Four slices of bacon, cut in half

Directions:
- ➢ Preheat the oven carefully to 350°F (175 degrees C).
- ➢ Combine the olive oil, Worcestershire sauce, turmeric, mustard, and garlic in a mixing bowl.
- ➢ Place the chicken breast halves in a medium baking dish and top with two bacon halves. Apply the glaze using a brush.
- ➢ Bake for 45 minutes, covered, in a preheated oven. Remove the lid and bake for another 15 minutes, or until the chicken juices run clear.

Chicken Rotini Soup

Preparation Time: 10 minutes
Cooking Time: 15 minutes
Servings: 1

Ingredients:

- 2 cubes chicken bouillon
- 1 (12 ounces) package of rotini pasta
- 13 cups of chicken broth
- 4 cups water
- Six stalks of celery, chopped
- One onion, chopped
- Four medium (blank)s carrots, chopped
- 1 ½ pounds chicken - cut into bite-size pieces
- garlic powder to taste
- One teaspoon of onion powder
- salt and pepper to taste

Directions:
- ➢ Boil the pasta in a 5-litre saucepan of water over high heat. Bring the bouillon to a boil in the water. Cook the rotini according to package directions in boiling water. Drain and put aside the pasta.
- ➢ Combine the chicken broth and water in a large saucepan over high heat. Add the celery, onion, carrots, and chicken to this. Bring to a boil, then add the reserved spaghetti. Reduce the heat to medium-low, cover, and season to taste with garlic powder, onion powder, and salt and pepper. Cook for 20 minutes, or until the veggies are soft and the chicken is no longer pink in the centre. Serve immediately.

Grilled Chicken and Herbs

Preparation Time: 10 minutes
Cooking Time: 15 minutes
Servings: 1

Ingredients:
- Four large skinless, boneless chicken breast halves
- Two tablespoons of olive oil
- One teaspoon of dried rosemary
- One teaspoon of dried thyme
- One teaspoon of dried oregano
- One teaspoon of chopped garlic
- ½ teaspoon salt
- ½ teaspoon ground black pepper

Directions:
- ➢ Preheat the grill to medium-high heat and liberally oil the grill grate.
- ➢ Rinse the chicken breasts and blot them dry with paper towels before piercing them many times with a fork. Pour olive oil over the chicken breasts in a large resealable plastic bag. Shut and shake the bag to coat the chicken in olive oil; add rosemary, thyme, oregano, garlic, salt, and black pepper to the bag, seal, and shake again to coat the chicken in herbs.
- ➢ Grill chicken breasts until the juices flow clear and an instant-read meat thermometer placed into the thickest part of the meat reads at least 160 degrees F (70 degrees C, about 10 minutes on each side) over a hot grill.

Chicken Soup

Preparation Time: 10 minutes
Cooking Time: 15 minutes
Servings: 1

Ingredients:
- One boneless chicken breast half, cooked and diced
- 2 cups water
- Two carrots, chopped
- One zucchini, diced
- One clove of garlic, minced
- ½ teaspoon chicken broth base

Directions:
- ➤ Bring cooked chicken flesh and water to a boil in a big saucepan.
- ➤ Cook for 5 to 10 minutes, then add the carrots, zucchini, and garlic.
- ➤ Cook for 5 minutes more after adding the chicken broth. Serve.

Italian Chicken Cacciatore
Preparation Time: 10 minutes
Cooking Time: 15 minutes
Servings: 1

Ingredients:
- ¼ cup olive oil, divided
- One onion, diced
- ¼ cup all-purpose flour
- ½ teaspoon salt
- ¼ teaspoon freshly ground black pepper
- Eight chicken thighs
- ½ cup dry white wine
- 2 (14.5 ounces) cans of diced tomatoes
- Two teaspoons of tomato paste
- ¼ teaspoon white sugar, or more to taste
- salt and ground black pepper to taste
- ½ cup chicken broth, or more as needed
- ½ cup black olives pitted
- One tablespoon of chopped fresh parsley
- One tablespoon of torn basil leaves

Directions:
- ➤ Heat two tablespoons of olive oil and saute onion in a pan over medium heat, frequently moving, until tender and translucent, about 5 minutes—place in a pot.
- ➤ In a large mixing bowl, combine flour, 1/2 teaspoon salt, and 1/4 teaspoon pepper. Toss the chicken thighs in the flour mixture to coat evenly.
- ➤ Heat the remaining two tablespoons of olive oil in a pan over medium heat, then add the chicken thighs and brown on one side for 5 minutes without flipping. Cook until the opposite side is browned, approximately 5 minutes more. Place the browned chicken thighs in the pot.
- ➤ Bring the white wine to a boil in the skillet. Stir to incorporate all of the browned chunks of chicken and flavours from the skillet into the soup. Season with salt and pepper, then add the chopped tomatoes, tomato paste, and sugar. Add enough chicken stock to cover the chicken. Cook, covered, over medium heat for 45 minutes, or until the chicken is no longer pink in the centre.
- ➤ Add the olives, parsley, and basil and mix well. Stir to heat thoroughly.

Fried Chicken
Preparation Time: 10 minutes
Cooking Time: 15 minutes
Servings: 1

Ingredients:
- 1 (4 pounds) chicken, cut into pieces
- salt and pepper to taste
- 1 ½ cups all-purpose flour for coating
- 2 quarts of vegetable oil for frying

Directions:
- ➤ Heat the oil in a large skillet over medium heat. Season the chicken pieces with salt and pepper to taste, then roll in flour to coat. Cook the chicken in a pan over medium heat until one side is golden brown, then flip and brown the other side until the chicken is no longer pink inside and the juices run clear. Drain on a paper towel before serving!

Chicken Yakisoba
Preparation Time: 10 minutes

Cooking Time: 15 minutes
Servings: 1

Ingredients:
- Two tablespoons of canola oil
- One tablespoon of sesame oil
- Two skinless, boneless chicken breast halves - cut into bite-size pieces
- Two cloves of garlic, minced
- Two tablespoons of Asian-style chile paste
- ½ cup soy sauce
- One tablespoon of canola oil
- ½ medium head cabbage, thinly sliced
- One onion, sliced
- Two carrots, cut into matchsticks
- One tablespoon salt
- 2 pounds cooked yakisoba noodles
- Two tablespoons pickled ginger, or to taste (Optional)

Directions:
- ➤ Heat two tablespoons of canola oil in a large pan and two tablespoons of sesame oil over medium-high heat. Cook and stir chicken and garlic in heated oil for 1 minute or until aromatic. Cook and stir the chile paste into the chicken mixture for 3 to 4 minutes, or until the chicken is thoroughly browned. Cook for 2 minutes after adding the soy sauce. Combine the chicken and sauce in a mixing basin.
- ➤ Heat one tablespoon of canola oil in a pan over medium-high heat; cook and stir cabbage, onion, carrots, and salt until cabbage is wilted, 3 to 4 minutes.
- ➤ Combine the chicken and cabbage mixtures. Cook and stir until the noodles are heated and the chicken is no longer pink on the inside, 3 to 4 minutes. Garnish with pickled ginger if desired.

Juicy Chicken
Preparation Time: 10 minutes
Cooking Time: 15 minutes
Servings: 1

Ingredients:
- ½ cup soy sauce
- ½ cup sherry or white cooking wine
- ½ cup chicken broth
- ¼ teaspoon ground ginger
- One pinch of garlic powder
- One bunch of green onions, chopped
- 1 pound skinless, boneless chicken breast halves - cut into 2 inch pieces

Directions:
- ➤ Combine the soy sauce, sherry, chicken broth, ginger, garlic powder, and green onions in a small pot. Bring to a boil, then remove from the heat. Place aside.
- ➤ Preheat the broiler in your oven. Thread chicken chunks onto skewers made of metal or bamboo. Place on a broiler pan that's been sprayed with cooking spray. 1 or 2 teaspoons of the sauce should be spooned over each chicken skewer.
- ➤ Place the pan in the broiler for 3 minutes or until browned. Remove from the oven, flip each, and spread additional sauce on top. Return to the oven until the chicken is well cooked and attractively browned.

Creamy Chicken and Noodles
Preparation Time: 10 minutes
Cooking Time: 15 minutes
Servings: 1

Ingredients:
- 1 (16 ounces) package of egg noodles
- ¼ cup butter
- ¼ cup chopped onion

- One tablespoon of minced garlic
- Six tablespoons of all-purpose flour
- 1 cup milk
- 1 cup half-and-half
- 30 ounces chicken broth
- 1 (3 pounds) rotisserie chicken, bones removed and meat cut into bite-size pieces
- 1 cup sour cream
- salt and ground black pepper to taste

Directions:
- ➢ Warm up a big saucepan of gently salted water. Cook egg noodles in boiling water for 5 minutes, tossing regularly, until cooked through yet firm to the biting. Transfer to a large serving dish after draining.
- ➢ Melt butter in a large saucepan over medium heat; cook and stir onion and garlic in the hot butter for 5 minutes, or until onion is transparent. Shake the flour, milk, and half-and-half in a jar with a lid until the flour is evenly combined with the milk and half-and-half. Pour mixture into skillet and stir for 5 minutes, or until smooth and thick.
- ➢ Whisk in the chicken broth gradually and bring to a boil, stirring constantly. To serve, stir cooked chicken and sour cream into sauce, season with salt and black pepper, and combine with cooked noodles.

Shoyu Chicken
Preparation Time: 10 minutes
Cooking Time: 15 minutes
Servings: 1

Ingredients:
- 1 cup soy sauce
- 1 cup brown sugar
- 1 cup water
- Four cloves of garlic, minced
- One onion, chopped
- One tablespoon grated fresh ginger root
- One tablespoon of ground black pepper
- One tablespoon of dried oregano
- One teaspoon of crushed red pepper flakes (optional)
- One teaspoon of ground cayenne pepper (Optional)
- One teaspoon of ground paprika (Optional)
- 5 pounds of skinless chicken thighs

Directions:
- ➢ In a large glass or ceramic mixing bowl, combine the soy sauce, brown sugar, water, garlic, onion, ginger, black pepper, oregano, red pepper flakes, cayenne pepper, and paprika. Toss in the chicken thighs to coat evenly. Cover the bowl with plastic wrap and refrigerate the chicken for at least 1 hour.
- ➢ Preheat an outside grill to medium heat and grease the grate liberally.
- ➢ Take the chicken thighs out of the marinade. Remove and discard the leftover marinade. Grill the chicken thighs until cooked through, about 15 minutes on each side, on a preheated grill.

Chinese Garlic Chicken
Preparation Time: 10 minutes
Cooking Time: 15 minutes
Servings: 1

Ingredients:
- 1 ½ pound skinless, boneless chicken breasts
- One teaspoon salt
- ½ teaspoon black pepper
- Two tablespoons of all-purpose flour
- Two tablespoons of peanut oil
- 15 cloves garlic, peeled
- Three tablespoons Shao-Hsing cooking wine or dry sherry
- Two tablespoons of light soy sauce
- One ⅓ cup of chicken stock

Directions:
- ➢ Season the chicken with salt and pepper. Toss in the flour until evenly covered.
- ➢ Heat the peanut oil over high heat in a wok or big pan until it begins to smoke. Stir in the chicken and cook for 3 to 5 minutes, or until the chunks are lightly browned on the exterior. Turn the heat to medium and add the entire garlic cloves, constantly stirring for 5 minutes.
- ➢ Reduce the heat to low and stir in the Shao-Hsing wine, soy sauce, and chicken stock. Cook, covered, for 20 minutes, or until the chicken is cooked. Before serving, remove the garlic cloves.

Buffalo Chicken Sauce
Preparation Time: 10 minutes
Cooking Time: 15 minutes
Servings: 1

Ingredients:
- 1 ½ cups butter
- 1 (12 fluid ounce) can or bottle of hot sauce

Directions:
- ➢ Melt butter in a small saucepan over medium heat or in a microwave on high for 30 seconds. Remove the white foam from the top and stir in the spicy sauce. Remove from the heat and put aside until the mixture begins to solidify.

Curried Chicken
Preparation Time: 10 minutes
Cooking Time: 15 minutes
Servings: 1

Ingredients:
- One whole chicken
- salt and ground black pepper to taste
- One tablespoon paprika, or to taste
- One tablespoon butter
- One apple, cored and chopped
- One onion, chopped
- One tablespoon curry powder, or more to taste
- 1 (10.75 ounces) can of cream of mushroom soup
- 1 cup half-and-half cream

Directions:
- ➢ Preheat the oven carefully to 350°F (175 degrees C).
- ➢ In a 9x13-inch baking dish, arrange the chicken pieces in a single layer. Set aside. Season the chicken well with salt, pepper, and paprika.
- ➢ In a pan over medium heat, melt the butter. Add the apple and onion to the melted butter, season with curry powder, and simmer and stir for 7 to 10 minutes, or until the apple and onion are soft. Stir in the mushroom soup and half-and-half until well blended; spoon over the chicken pieces.
- ➢ Bake for 75 minutes, or until the meat is no longer pink at the bone and the juices flow clear. An instant-read thermometer implanted near the bone into the thickest section of the thigh should register 180 degrees F. (82 degrees C).

Dilly Chicken
Preparation Time: 10 minutes
Cooking Time: 15 minutes
Servings: 1

Ingredients:
- 3 pounds of bone-in chicken pieces
- 1 (10.75 ounces) can of condensed cream of mushroom soup
- 1 cup milk
- 1 cup sour cream
- One teaspoon of dry onion soup mix
- One teaspoon of dried dill weed

Directions:

- ➢ Preheat the oven carefully to 350° F. (175 degrees C). Grease a 9x13-inch baking dish with cooking spray.
- ➢ Place the chicken pieces in the baking dish that has been prepared. Pour the undiluted mushroom soup, milk, and sour cream over the chicken—season with dill and onion soup mix. There is no need to stir.
- ➢ Bake for 1 1/2 hours, or until the chicken falls from the bone, in a preheated oven. The longer you can let it cook, the better it will taste.

Cheesy Chicken Spaghetti

Preparation Time: 10 minutes
Cooking Time: 15 minutes
Servings: 1

Ingredients:
- Two tablespoons of salted butter
- 1 (8 ounces) package of sliced fresh mushrooms
- One medium red bell pepper, diced
- 2 pounds skinless, boneless chicken breasts
- 1 (23 ounces) can of condensed cream of mushroom soup
- 1 (14 ounces) can of diced tomatoes, drained
- One tablespoon of Worcestershire sauce
- Two teaspoons of seasoned salt
- Three cloves of garlic, minced
- 1 (8 ounces) package of shredded sharp Cheddar cheese
- 1 (8 ounces) package of cream cheese
- 1 (16 ounces) package of spaghetti

Directions:
- ➢ In a pan over medium-high heat, melt the butter. Sauté the mushrooms and bell pepper for 3 minutes, or until a soft—place in a slow cooker.
- ➢ Place the chicken in the slow cooker. Combine condensed soup, chopped tomatoes, Worcestershire sauce, seasoned salt, and garlic in a mixing bowl. Cook, covered, for 3 1/2 hours on Low or 2 hours on High, or until the chicken is no longer pink in the middle and the juices flow clear. In the middle, an instant-read thermometer should read at least 165 degrees F. (74 degrees C). Remove the chicken and set aside for 5 minutes, or until cool enough to handle.
- ➢ In the slow cooker, combine the Cheddar and cream cheese. Return the chilled chicken to the slow cooker and shred with two forks. Cook until the cheese has melted, about 10 to 15 minutes on High.
- ➢ Meanwhile, heat a big pot of gently salted water. Cook the spaghetti in boiling water for 12 minutes, tossing periodically until cooked yet firm to the biting. Drain and place in the slow cooker. Serve with a stir.

Easy Chicken Marsala

Preparation Time: 10 minutes
Cooking Time: 15 minutes
Servings: 1

Ingredients:
- Three tablespoons of olive oil
- ⅓ cup heavy cream
- 1 cup sliced fresh mushrooms
- 4 (6 ounces) skinless, boneless chicken breast halves
- ¼ cup chopped green onion
- salt and pepper to taste
- ⅓ cup Marsala wine
- ⅛ cup milk

Directions:
- ➢ In a large pan over medium heat, heat the olive oil. Cook chicken in heated oil for 15 to 20 minutes, or until cooked through and juices flow clear.
- ➢ Sauté the mushrooms and green onions in the pan until tender, then add the Marsala wine and bring to a boil.
- ➢ Continue to boil for 2 to 4 minutes, adjusting to taste with salt and pepper. Stir in the cream and milk and cook for 5 minutes, or until well cooked.

Happy Roast Chicken

Preparation Time: 10 minutes
Cooking Time: 15 minutes
Servings: 1

Ingredients:
- ½ cup dry white wine
- Two lemons, cut in half
- Six large cloves of garlic
- 1 (4 pounds) whole chicken
- 1 ½ teaspoon cold butter
- Two tablespoons of Dijon mustard
- salt and pepper

Directions:
- ➢ Preheat the oven carefully to 425°F (220 degrees C). Set aside the wine in a 10-inch cast-iron skillet.
- ➢ Insert the lemon halves and garlic cloves into the chicken cavity. Half of the butter should be slid underneath the skin of each breast. Rub the Dijon mustard all over the chicken, then season with salt & pepper to taste. Place the cast-iron skillet on top.
- ➢ Bake the chicken for 15 minutes at 350 degrees F (175 degrees C), decrease the heat to 350 degrees F (175 degrees C), and continue baking until the chicken is no longer pink at the bone and the juices flow clear, about 1 hour more. An instant-read thermometer implanted near the bone into the thickest section of the thigh should register 180 degrees F. (82 degrees C). Remove the chicken from the oven, cover with a doubled layer of aluminium foil, and set aside for 15 minutes to rest before slicing.

Cheesy Chicken Spaghetti

Preparation Time: 10 minutes
Cooking Time: 15 minutes
Servings: 1

Ingredients:
- Two tablespoons of salted butter
- 1 (8 ounces) package of sliced fresh mushrooms
- One medium red bell pepper, diced
- 2 pounds skinless, boneless chicken breasts
- 1 (23 ounces) can of condensed cream of mushroom soup
- 1 (14 ounces) can of diced tomatoes, drained
- One tablespoon of Worcestershire sauce
- Two teaspoons of seasoned salt
- Three cloves of garlic, minced
- 1 (8 of an ounce) package of shredded sharp Cheddar cheese
- 1 (8 ounces) package of cream cheese
- 1 (16 ounces) package of spaghetti

Directions:
- ➢ In a pan over medium-high heat, melt the butter. Sauté the mushrooms and bell pepper for 3 minutes, or until a soft—place in a slow cooker.
- ➢ Place the chicken in the slow cooker. Combine condensed soup, chopped tomatoes, Worcestershire sauce, seasoned salt, and garlic in a mixing bowl. Cook, covered, for 3 1/2 hours on Low or 2 hours on High, or until the chicken is no longer pink in the middle and the juices flow clear. In the middle, an instant-read thermometer should read at least 165 degrees F. (74 degrees C). Remove the chicken and set aside for 5 minutes, or until cool enough to handle.
- ➢ In the slow cooker, combine the Cheddar and cream cheese. Return the chilled chicken to the slow cooker and shred with two forks. Cook until the cheese has melted, about 10 to 15 minutes on High.
- ➢ Meanwhile, heat a big pot of gently salted water. Cook the spaghetti in boiling water for 12 minutes, tossing periodically until cooked yet firm to the biting. Drain and place in the slow cooker. Serve with a stir.

Easy Chicken Marsala

Preparation Time: 10 minutes
Cooking Time: 15 minutes
Servings: 1

Ingredients:

- Three tablespoons of olive oil
- 1 cup sliced fresh mushrooms
- 4 (6 ounces) skinless, boneless chicken breast halves
- ⅓ cup heavy cream
- ⅓ cup Marsala wine
- ¼ cup chopped green onion, salt and pepper to taste
- ⅛ cup milk

Directions:

➢ In a large pan over medium heat, heat the olive oil. Cook chicken in heated oil for 15 to 20 minutes, or until cooked through and juices flow clear.

➢ Sauté the mushrooms and green onions in the pan until tender, then add the Marsala wine and bring to a boil.

➢ Continue to boil for 2 to 4 minutes, adjusting to taste with salt and pepper. Stir in the cream and milk and cook for 5 minutes, or until well cooked.

CHAPTER 15: MEAT

Kale Lasagna with Meat Sauce

Preparation Time: 10 minutes
Cooking Time: 15 minutes
Servings: 1

Ingredients:
- 1 pound Italian pork sausage, casings removed
- 1 pound of ground beef
- ½ cup minced onion
- Two cloves of garlic, crushed
- 1 (14.5 ounces) can of crushed tomatoes
- 2 (6 ounces) cans of tomato paste
- ½ cup vegetable broth
- Two tablespoons of Italian seasoning
- salt and ground black pepper to taste
- 1 (16 ounces) package of lasagna noodles
- 1 (16 ounces) container of ricotta cheese
- 2 cups chopped kale
- One egg
- 1 cup grated Parmesan cheese
- 1 pound shredded mozzarella cheese

Directions:
- ➤ Preheat the oven carefully to 375° F. (190 degrees C).
- ➤ In a large saucepan over medium-high heat, brown and stir Italian sausage, ground beef, onion, and garlic until meats are browned and crumbly, 5 to 7 minutes. Crush the tomatoes, and add the tomato paste, vegetable broth, Italian spice, salt, and pepper to taste. Bring to a low boil. Reduce the heat to low and cook, stirring periodically, for about 1 hour.
- ➤ Meanwhile, heat a big pot of gently salted water. Cook the lasagna noodles in boiling water for 8 minutes, tossing periodically, until soft yet firm to the biting.
- ➤ Combine the ricotta cheese, kale, and egg in a mixing dish.
- ➤ Layer the lasagna in a 9x13-inch baking dish, beginning with a small amount of meat sauce and noodles, then 1/2 of the ricotta mixture, more noodles, then the majority of the remaining meat sauce. Continue with the remaining Parmesan cheese, 1/2 of the mozzarella cheese, noodles, remaining ricotta mixture, and meat sauce. Finish with the remaining mozzarella cheese.
- ➤ 30 to 45 minutes bake uncovered in a warm oven until bubbling and golden. Allow 10 minutes to cool and solidify before cutting.

Blue Cheese, Spinach Meat Loaf Muffins

Preparation Time: 10 minutes
Cooking Time: 15 minutes
Servings: 1

Ingredients:
- 1 ½ pounds lean ground beef
- ¾ cup crumbled blue cheese
- ½ cup diced onion
- ½ cup Italian bread crumbs
- ½ cup chopped fresh spinach
- Two eggs
- Two tablespoons of Worcestershire sauce

Directions:
- ➤ Preheat the oven carefully to 375°F (190 degrees C). Cooking spray should be sprayed into a big muffin tin.
- ➤ In a large mixing bowl, combine ground beef, blue cheese, onion, bread crumbs, spinach, eggs, and Worcestershire sauce until thoroughly combined. Divide the meat mixture equally among the prepared muffin cups.

- ➤ Thirty minutes in a preheated oven until the middle is no longer pink. In the middle, an instant-read thermometer should read at least 160 degrees F. (70 degrees C).

Syrian Rice with Meat

Preparation Time: 10 minutes
Cooking Time: 15 minutes
Servings: 1

Ingredients:
- ¼ cup butter
- 2 pounds of ground beef
- Two teaspoons salt
- ½ teaspoon ground allspice
- ½ teaspoon ground cinnamon
- ½ teaspoon ground black pepper
- 4 ½ cups chicken broth
- 2 cups long-grain white rice
- Two tablespoons butter
- ½ cup pine nuts

Directions:
- ➤ In a large saucepan over medium-high heat, melt 1/4 cup butter. Mix in the ground meat, salt, allspice, cinnamon, and black pepper—Cook for 7 to 10 minutes, or until the meat is browned.
- ➤ Pour in the chicken broth and rice. Bring to a boil, covered. Cook until the liquid has been absorbed, about 20 minutes.
- ➤ Meanwhile, melt two tablespoons of butter in a small pan over medium heat. Cook until the pine nuts are gently toasted, 3 to 5 minutes.
- ➤ Before serving, toss pine nuts into the rice and meat combination.

Deer Meat

Preparation Time: 10 minutes
Cooking Time: 15 minutes
Servings: 1

Ingredients:
- 1 ½ pounds venison (deer meat)
- Two onions, chopped
- 4 cups fresh mushrooms, sliced
- Three tablespoons butter
- One clove of garlic, minced
- 1 (6 ounces) can of tomato paste
- One teaspoon of all-purpose flour
- 1 cup sour cream
- One teaspoon salt
- One pinch of mustard powder
- ⅛ teaspoon dried parsley

Directions:
- ➤ In a large pan over medium heat, melt butter or margarine. Sauté the onions till transparent, then add the meat and brown it.
- ➤ After gently browning the meat, add mushrooms, garlic, tomato paste, flour, sour cream, salt, mustard powder, and parsley. Stir everything together, then decrease the heat to low and let it simmer for 20 to 30 minutes. The longer it cooks, the softer the flesh becomes. Enjoy!

Sicilian Meat Roll

Preparation Time: 10 minutes
Cooking Time: 15 minutes
Servings: 1

Ingredients:

- Two eggs, beaten
- ½ cup tomato juice
- ¾ cup soft bread crumbs
- Two tablespoons of snipped fresh parsley
- ½ teaspoon dried oregano, crushed
- ¼ teaspoon sea salt
- ¼ teaspoon ground black pepper
- One clove of garlic, minced
- 2 pounds lean ground beef
- 1 (6 ounces) package of thinly sliced ham
- 1 (6 ounces) package of sliced mozzarella cheese

Directions:

- Combine the eggs and tomato juice in a large mixing basin. Combine the bread crumbs, parsley, oregano, salt, pepper, garlic, and ground beef in a mixing bowl. Thoroughly combine—Preheat the oven carefully to 350°F (175 degrees C).
- Pat and shape the meat into a 10x8 inch rectangle on a piece of foil or waxed paper. Place ham slices on the meat, leaving a border around the edges. Tear up the cheese pieces, leaving one whole, and scatter over the ham.
- Gently wrap up the meat, lifting with foil or waxed paper starting from the short end. Seal the meat's edges and ends. Place the roll in a 9x13 inch baking dish, seam side down.
- Bake for 75 minutes in a preheated oven. Cut the reserved cheese slice into four triangles. Place the triangles on top of the bread—Bake for a further 2 minutes, or until the cheese melts.

Monkey Meat

Preparation Time: 10 minutes
Cooking Time: 15 minutes
Servings: 1

Ingredients:

- 4 pounds tri-tip roast
- Three teaspoons of salt, divided
- ¾ teaspoon ground black pepper, divided
- Three tablespoons chilli powder, divided
- Three tablespoons of ground cumin, divided
- ⅓ cup olive oil, divided
- Two large onions, chopped
- Four cloves of garlic, chopped
- 2 Anaheim chile peppers, chopped
- One poblano chile pepper, chopped
- Two jalapeno chile peppers, chopped
- One green bell pepper, seeded and chopped
- One carrot, chopped
- Two stalks of celery, chopped
- Four Roma (plum) tomatoes, chopped
- One whole dried red chile pepper, seeded and chopped
- 1 (14 ounces) can of beef broth

Directions:

- Remove the extra fat and tissue from the beef roast and chop it into 4 or 5 big portions. 2 teaspoons salt, 1/2 teaspoon pepper, one tablespoon chilli powder, and one tablespoon crushed cumin in a cup or small bowl. Rub this mixture into the meat and set it aside for 15 minutes at room temperature.
- In a large deep pan or Dutch oven, heat three tablespoons of olive oil. All sides of the meat should be seared. Remove the meat from the pan and drizzle with the remaining olive oil. Reduce the heat to medium and stir in the onions, garlic, Anaheim peppers, poblano peppers, jalapeno peppers, green pepper, carrot, and celery. Cook for about 5 minutes, stirring periodically, to allow the flavours to come together.
- Season the Roma tomatoes with the remaining chilli powder, cumin, salt, pepper, and dried chile pepper in the pan—Cook for 5 minutes on low heat.

- Stir in the beef broth and return the meat to the pan. Bring to a boil, then reduce to low heat and cook for 3 to 3 1/2 hours, or until the meat is very soft—season with salt and pepper to taste. Remove the meat from the saucepan, shred it, and return it to the pot. If necessary, reheat before serving.

Layered Taco Dip with Meat

Preparation Time: 10 minutes
Cooking Time: 15 minutes
Servings: 1

Ingredients:

- 1 pound of ground beef
- 2 (1.25 ounce) packages of mild taco seasoning mix (such as McCormick®), divided
- 1 (16 ounces) container of sour cream
- 1 (8 ounces) package of cream cheese
- 1 (8 ounces) package of shredded Cheddar cheese, divided
- 1 (16 ounces) package of shredded lettuce
- 1 (8 ounces) jar salsa, or to taste

Directions:

- Melt butter in a large pan over medium-high heat. Cook and stir meat in a heated pan for 5 to 7 minutes, or until browned and crumbly; season with one box of taco seasoning mix. Grease should be drained and discarded. Allow the meat to cool fully.
- Combine the sour cream, cream cheese, and remaining taco spice mix in a mixing bowl until smooth.
- Cover a baking sheet with the sour cream mixture. Sprinkle half of the Cheddar cheese equally over the sour cream layer; top with the ground beef, lettuce, and remaining Cheddar cheese, in that order. Pour the salsa over the dip.
- Refrigerate for at least one hour.

Polish Meat and Potatoes

Preparation Time: 10 minutes
Cooking Time: 15 minutes
Servings: 1

Ingredients:

- Four potatoes, peeled and cut into 1-inch cubes
- One onion, chopped
- Two green bell peppers, cut into 1-inch pieces
- ½ teaspoon onion powder
- ½ teaspoon garlic powder
- ½ teaspoon salt
- ¼ teaspoon black pepper
- ¼ cup vegetable oil
- 1 (16 ounces) package of kielbasa sausage, cut into 1-inch pieces

Directions:

- In a large skillet over medium-high heat, heat the oil. Cook, stirring periodically, for 15 minutes with the onions and potatoes. Reduce the heat to medium and add the bell pepper, onion powder, garlic powder, salt, and pepper to taste. Cook for 5 minutes, covered. Cover and heat for 15 minutes, or until the onions are caramelized.

Taco Meat

Preparation Time: 10 minutes
Cooking Time: 15 minutes
Servings: 1

Ingredients:

- 1 pound lean ground beef
- ½ teaspoon onion powder
- ½ teaspoon garlic salt
- ½ teaspoon celery salt
- ½ teaspoon ground cumin
- 1 (8 ounces) can tomato sauce, or more to taste

Directions:
- ➤ Melt butter in a large pan over medium-high heat. 5 to 7 minutes, cook and toss the meat in a heated pan until browned and crumbly.
- ➤ Onion powder, garlic salt, celery salt, and cumin season the meat. Pour the tomato sauce over the meat, swirl to moisten, and cook until slightly thickened, about 5 minutes.

Alysia's Basic Meat Lasagna
Preparation Time: 10 minutes
Cooking Time: 15 minutes
Servings: 1

Ingredients:
- 1 ½ pounds ground beef
- One teaspoon of garlic powder
- 1 (28 ounces) jar sausage flavoured spaghetti sauce
- 1 (8 ounces) can of tomato sauce
- One teaspoon of dried oregano
- One tablespoon of olive oil
- Four cloves of garlic, minced
- One small onion, diced
- 1 (8 ounces) package of mozzarella cheese, shredded
- 8 ounces provolone cheese, shredded
- 1 (15 ounces) container of ricotta cheese
- Two eggs
- ¼ cup milk
- ½ teaspoon dried oregano
- Nine lasagna noodles
- ¼ cup grated Parmesan cheese

Directions:
- ➤ Preheat the oven carefully to 375°F (190 degrees C).
- ➤ Garlic powder is used to season ground beef. Melt butter in a large pan over medium-high heat. Cook and stir ground beef in a heated pan for 5 to 7 minutes, or until browned and crumbly. Grease should be drained and discarded.
- ➤ Combine the spaghetti sauce, tomato sauce, and oregano in a large pot. Place aside.
- ➤ In a large pan over medium-high heat, heat the olive oil. Cook until the garlic and onions are cooked and transparent, about 5 minutes. Incorporate the sautéed onion-garlic combination and ground beef into the sauce mixture. Allow simmering for 15 to 20 minutes, covered.
- ➤ In a medium mixing bowl, combine the mozzarella and provolone cheeses. Combine the ricotta cheese, eggs, milk, and 1/2 teaspoon of oregano in a separate dish.
- ➤ Fill a 9x13-inch baking pan halfway with sauce to cover the bottom. Place three lasagna noodles on top of the sauce in the pan. Cover with additional sauce, then ricotta mixture, then mozzarella/provolone combination; layer again. Finish with a layer of noodles and any leftover sauce. Top with the Parmesan cheese.
- ➤ Bake for 30 minutes, covered, in a preheated oven. Uncover and bake for another 15 minutes until the cheese has melted and the top is brown.

Meat Pie
Preparation Time: 10 minutes
Cooking Time: 15 minutes
Servings: 1

Ingredients:
- One medium potato, peeled and cubed
- ½ pound ground beef
- ½ pound ground pork
- ⅓ clove garlic, chopped
- ½ cup chopped onion
- ¼ cup water
- ½ teaspoon mustard powder
- ½ teaspoon dried thyme
- ¼ teaspoon ground cloves
- One teaspoon salt

- ¼ teaspoon ground black pepper
- ¼ teaspoon dried sage
- 1 package of refrigerated pie crusts

Directions:
- ➤ Preheat the oven carefully to 425° F. (220 degrees C). Place the potato in a saucepan and cover with water. Bring to a boil and simmer for 5 minutes, or until the potatoes are cooked. Set aside after draining and mashing.
- ➤ Meanwhile, in a large saucepan, combine the ground beef and pork with the garlic, onion, and water—season with salt, mustard powder, thyme, and cloves. Cook, tossing to crumble the meat and mix in the spices over medium heat until the meat is uniformly browned. Take the pan off the heat and stir in the mashed potatoes.
- ➤ Fill a 9-inch pie pan with one of the pie crusts. Fill with the meat mixture and top with the remaining pie crust. To release steam, prick the top crust several times with a knife. Remove any extra dough by crimping over the edges with the tines of a fork. Wrap aluminium foil around the pie crust's edges.
- ➤ Bake for 25 minutes, or until the crust is golden brown, in a preheated oven. Serve alone or with beef gravy.

Good Old Meat Pie
Preparation Time: 10 minutes
Cooking Time: 15 minutes
Servings: 1

Ingredients:
- One recipe pastry for a 9-inch single-crust pie
- Three tablespoons margarine
- ½ cup chopped onion
- One potato, diced
- ⅓ cup all-purpose flour
- ½ teaspoon dried oregano
- ½ teaspoon garlic powder
- ¼ teaspoon black pepper
- One ¼ cups beef broth
- One carrot, chopped
- 1 cup frozen green peas
- 2 cups cubed cooked or leftover beef

Directions:
- ➤ Preheat the oven carefully to 425° F. (220 degrees C). Roll out the pie dough into a 12-inch circle on a lightly floured board. Place aside.
- ➤ In a saucepan over medium heat, melt the margarine. Cook the potato and onion until the onion is soft but not brown. Pour the flour over the mixture and whisk to combine. Add oregano, black pepper, and garlic powder to taste. Add the peas, carrot, and meat after pouring the beef broth. Bring the water to a boil. Place the pastry over the top of the mixture in a 2-quart casserole dish. Make steam slits and flute the edges.
- ➤ Bake for 25 to 30 minutes, or until the crust is brown, on a baking sheet. Allow thickening for 10 minutes before serving.

Halloween Meat Head
Preparation Time: 10 minutes
Cooking Time: 15 minutes
Servings: 1

Ingredients:
- life-sized decorative plastic skull
- 1 (8 ounces) package of cream cheese, softened
- 1 pound thinly sliced deli ham, or as needed

Directions:
- ➤ A plastic skull should be washed and dried—smear cream cheese on the skull.
- ➤ Cover the skull with a single layer of ham, leaving the eyes and fangs exposed.

Argentine Meat Empanadas

Preparation Time: 10 minutes
Cooking Time: 15 minutes
Servings: 1

Ingredients:

- ½ cup shortening
- Two onions, chopped
- 1 pound lean ground beef
- Two teaspoons of Hungarian sweet paprika
- ¾ teaspoon hot paprika
- ½ teaspoon crushed red pepper flakes
- One teaspoon of ground cumin
- One tablespoon of distilled white vinegar
- ¼ cup raisins
- ½ cup pitted green olives, chopped
- Two hard-cooked eggs, chopped
- salt to taste
- 1 (17.5 ounces) package of frozen puff pastry sheets, thawed

Directions:

- ➢ Melt the shortening in a sauté pan and add the chopped onions. Cook the onions until they are just starting to turn yellow. Stir in the sweet paprika, spicy paprika, crushed red pepper flakes, and salt to taste.
- ➢ Pour boiling water over the meat in a colander to partially cook it. Allow the meat to cool completely. Place the meat on a plate and season with salt, cumin, and vinegar to taste. Combine the meat and onion mixture. Mix well and place on a flat plate to cool and solidify.
- ➢ Make ten circular shells out of puff pastry dough. Add a tablespoon of the meat mixture to each round, including some raisins, olives, and hard-boiled egg. Avoid getting the filling to the edges of the dough since the oiliness will hinder effective sealing. Wet the edge of the pastry, fold it in half, and adhere the edges together. The form should be similar to a 2/3 to 1/2 inch flat border of pastry to work with. Seal by twisting the edge between your thumb and index finger, adding pressure before releasing the pinch and going on to the next curl. Other sealing methods, such as pinching without curling or closing with a fork, will not prevent fluid leaks during baking because empanadas must be juicy.
- ➢ Preheat the oven carefully to 350°F (180 degrees C). Place the empanadas on a baking sheet lined with parchment paper. To let steam escape during baking, puncture each empanada with a fork at the curl. Bake until brown and glazed with egg, about 20 to 30 minutes.

Easter Meat Pie

Preparation Time: 10 minutes
Cooking Time: 15 minutes
Servings: 1

Ingredients:

- 4 (9 inches) unbaked pie crusts
- 2 pounds of ricotta cheese
- Six eggs
- 8 ounces mozzarella cheese, grated
- 1 pound cooked ham, chopped
- ½ pound Genoa salami, chopped
- ¼ pound prosciutto, chopped
- ¼ cup grated Parmesan cheese

Directions:

- ➢ Preheat the oven carefully to 325°F (165 degrees C).
- ➢ In a large mixing bowl, combine ricotta and eggs, one at a time, while mixing on low speed. Stir in the mozzarella, ham, salami, and prosciutto until completely blended—line two 9-inch baking pans with puff pastry. Half of the mixture should be placed in each pan. Sprinkle half of the Parmesan cheese over each pie before covering with the top dough. Crimp the edges and make steam vents at the tops.

- ➢ Bake for 1 hour, or until the crust is golden brown, in a preheated oven. Allow cooling on racks.

Natchitoches Meat Pies

Preparation Time: 10 minutes
Cooking Time: 15 minutes
Servings: 1

Ingredients:

- One tablespoon of vegetable oil
- One tablespoon of all-purpose flour
- One onion, chopped
- 1 pound bulk pork sausage
- 1 pound of ground beef
- One teaspoon of Cajun seasoning
- One pinch of garlic powder
- 1 (15 ounces) package of store-bought refrigerated pie dough, at room temperature
- 1-quart vegetable oil for deep frying

Directions:

- ➢ Heat one tablespoon oil in a large pan over medium-low heat; stir in flour and cook until flour goes from white to a nutty brown colour, 2 to 3 minutes. Cook until the onion is translucent, about 5 minutes. Brown the meats for 10 to 12 minutes, or until no longer pink; toss in Cajun spice and garlic powder; drain fat. Allow cooling to room temperature.
- ➢ Roll out the dough to 1/4 inch on a lightly floured board. Use a 5-inch diameter round cookie cutter or cut around a saucer to form a dough circle. Fill each round with a heaping scoop of meat filling. Fold the dough over the filling and press the edges tight with a fork or your fingertips. Repeat to produce 15 pies, rerolling scraps of dough as required.
- ➢ Heat the frying oil in a deep fryer to 375°F (190 degrees C).
- ➢ Deep-fried pies in small batches for 3 to 4 minutes, or until golden brown. Dry with paper towels. Alternatively, bake pies on prepared cookie sheets in a preheated 350°F (175°C) oven for 15 to 20 minutes, or until golden brown.

Basic Seitan - Wheat Meat (Vegan Meat Substitute)

Preparation Time: 10 minutes
Cooking Time: 15 minutes
Servings: 1

Ingredients:

- 1 cup vital wheat gluten
- Three tablespoons of nutritional yeast
- ½ cup vegetable broth
- ¼ cup liquid amino acid (such as Bragg®)
- One tablespoon of olive oil
- 1 ½ teaspoons minced garlic
- Cooking Broth:
- 4 cups vegetable broth
- 4 cups water
- ¼ cup tamari

Directions:

- ➢ In a mixing dish, combine vital wheat gluten, nutritional yeast, 1/2 cup vegetable broth, liquid amino acid, olive oil, and garlic until the ingredients form a ball. Knead the dough until it acquires a springy feel. Divide the dough into three equal halves and form into 1/2-inch thick patties.
- ➢ In a large saucepan, bring 4 cups of vegetable broth, water, and tamari to a boil. Place patties carefully into boiling stock; cover saucepan and bring to a boil. Reduce heat to low and set lid slightly askew to vent steam. Continue cooking patties until firm, approximately 1 hour, rotating patties regularly. Remove the saucepan from the heat and set the cover aside. Allow the patties to cool for 15 minutes in the broth before serving.

Nikujaga (Japanese-style meat and potatoes)

Preparation Time: 10 minutes
Cooking Time: 15 minutes
Servings: 1

Ingredients:

- Eight snow peas
- One tablespoon of vegetable oil
- ¼ pound sirloin steak, thinly sliced
- Four potatoes, cut into bite-sized pieces
- 2 cups dashi soup
- ¼ cup soy sauce
- ¼ cup sake
- One tablespoon of white sugar
- One onion, chopped

Directions:

- ➢ Put the snow peas in a small saucepan with enough water to cover; bring to a boil and remove from heat immediately. Set aside after draining.
- ➢ Heat the oil in a large skillet over medium heat; brown the meat in the oil. Cook and stir until the potatoes are tender, 5 to 7 minutes. Simmer for 10 minutes after adding the dashi soup, soy sauce, sake, and sugar.
- ➢ Reduce the heat to low and spread the chopped onion over the mixture; continue to simmer for another 15 minutes, or until the liquid has nearly totally evaporated. To serve, top the mixture with the snow peas.

Spicy Harissa Meat Pies

Preparation Time: 10 minutes
Cooking Time: 15 minutes
Servings: 1

Ingredients:

- 1 pound red chile peppers, chopped
- Five cloves of garlic, minced
- Four tablespoons of olive oil
- One tablespoon of Mexican chilli powder
- One teaspoon of ground coriander
- One teaspoon of ground cumin
- One teaspoon of dried lime granules
- ½ teaspoon sea salt
- Pastry:
- 2 cups unbleached all-purpose flour
- One tablespoon of hot chilli powder
- ½ tablespoon ground cumin
- ¼ teaspoon sea salt
- ¼ cup cold butter
- ¼ cup shortening (such as Crisco®)
- ⅓ cup cold, flat beer
- Three tablespoons of olive oil
- One large onion, minced
- Six large cloves of garlic, minced
- ½ pound lean ground beef
- ½ teaspoon salt
- ½ teaspoon freshly ground black pepper
- ½ teaspoon ground cumin
- ½ teaspoon dried thyme
- ½ cup bread crumbs
- ¼ cup beef stock
- Three teaspoons of Mexican chilli powder
- Two teaspoons of cayenne pepper
- ¼ cup cold, flat beer
- One egg, beaten

Directions:

- ➢ In a food processor, combine chile peppers, garlic, olive oil, chilli powder, coriander, cumin, lime granules, and sea salt; pulse until combined. Set aside 1/2 cup harissa and refrigerate the rest for another use.
- ➢ Step 2
- ➢ Combine the flour, chilli powder, cumin, and sea salt for the pastry in a food processor. Pulse in the butter and shorten until the mixture is crumbly. Pour in a little cold beer at a time, running the processor, until a ball of dough forms and pulls away from the edges.
- ➢ Roll the dough to about 1/8 inch on a lightly floured silicone pastry mat. While you make the meat filling, cut the dough into eight 8-inch circles and wrap it with waxed paper or a moist towel. (If refrigerating the dough overnight, set it out for at least 15 minutes before using.)
- ➢ In a big skillet over medium heat, heat the oil; add the onion and garlic—cook and stir for 5 minutes, or until the onion has softened and turned translucent. Combine the ground beef, salt, pepper, cumin, and thyme in a mixing bowl. Cook and stir for 10 minutes, or until the meat is browned and crumbly. Incorporate the reserved 1/2 cup harissa. Combine the bread crumbs, beef stock, chilli powder, and cayenne pepper in a mixing bowl. Cover and simmer, stirring periodically, for 10 to 15 minutes, or until all liquid has been absorbed and the filling is moist but not runny. Remove from the heat and leave to cool.
- ➢ Preheat the oven carefully to 400°F (200°C) and lightly butter a baking sheet.
- ➢ In a small dish, combine the beer and the egg.
- ➢ Uncover the dough circles and fill them with 2 to 3 tablespoons of the meat filling, leaving a clear margin of dough all the way around. Moisten the circular borders with the beer-egg mixture. Fold the dough in half, enclosing the filling, and seal the edges with a fork. Brush each pastry lightly with the beer-egg mixture and place on the prepared baking sheet.
- ➢ Bake for about 20 minutes, or until the pastries are golden brown.

Yummy Veal Meat Loaf

Preparation Time: 10 minutes
Cooking Time: 15 minutes
Servings: 1

Ingredients:

- 2 pounds ground veal
- 1 cup Italian seasoned bread crumbs
- One egg, beaten
- ⅓ cup shredded baby carrots
- 1 cup ketchup
- One tablespoon of chopped garlic
- ½ cup chopped onion
- One teaspoon salt
- One teaspoon of dried parsley
- ½ teaspoon chilli powder
- ½ teaspoon ground black pepper

Directions:

- ➢ Preheat the oven carefully to 375°F (190 degrees C).
- ➢ Combine the veal, bread crumbs, egg, baby carrots, 1/2 cup ketchup, garlic, and onion in a mixing bowl—season with salt, pepper, parsley, and chilli powder. Transfer to an 8x8-inch loaf pan and shape into a loaf. Finish with the remaining ketchup.
- ➢ Bake for 45 minutes, covered, in a preheated oven. Remove the top and bake for another 15 minutes, or until the internal temperature reaches 160 degrees F. (70 degrees C). Allow 10 minutes before serving.

CHAPTER 16: VEGETABLES

Beer Battered Fried Vegetables

Preparation Time: 10 minutes
Cooking Time: 15 minutes
Servings: 1

Ingredients:
- 2 cups all-purpose flour
- 1 ½ cups beer
- Two eggs
- 1 cup milk
- salt and pepper to taste
- 2 cups vegetable oil for frying
- One carrot, cut into thick strips
- One onion, sliced into rings
- Six fresh mushroom stems removed
- One green bell pepper, sliced in rings

Directions:
- ➤ Combine 1 1/2 cup flour and beer with a wooden spoon in a medium mixing basin; set aside at room temperature for at least 3 hours.
- ➤ In a small mixing dish, combine the eggs and milk. Combine 1/2 cup flour, salt, and pepper in a separate basin.
- ➤ Preheat the oil to 375°F (190 degrees C).
- ➤ Each veggie should be dipped in the egg and milk mixture. Next, dip the veggie in the flour and spice mixture, followed by the beer and flour combination. Fry the veggies in the oil until golden brown.

Grilled Vegetables with Balsamic Vinegar

Preparation Time: 10 minutes
Cooking Time: 15 minutes
Servings: 1

Ingredients:
- ½ cup olive oil
- Two tablespoons of soy sauce
- Two tablespoons of balsamic vinegar
- ½ teaspoon salt
- ½ teaspoon ground black pepper
- Two medium eggplants, cut into 1/2-inch slices
- Three medium zucchinis, cut into 1/2-inch slices
- Two medium green bell peppers, cut into 1/2-inch slices

Directions:
- ➤ Combine the olive oil, soy sauce, balsamic vinegar, salt, and pepper in a large mixing bowl. Marinate eggplant, zucchini, and bell peppers in soy sauce. Marinate for approximately 45 minutes.
- ➤ Preheat the grill to medium-high heat and liberally oil the grill grate. Shake off any extra marinade from the veggies.
- ➤ Grill veggies on a hot grill for 10 to 15 minutes, coating with marinade. Serve the cooked veggies with any residual marinade on a plate.

Marinated Barbequed Vegetables

Preparation Time: 10 minutes
Cooking Time: 15 minutes
Servings: 1

Ingredients:
- One small eggplant, cut into 3/4 inch thick slices
- Two small red bell peppers, seeded and cut into wide strips
- Three zucchinis, sliced
- Six fresh mushroom stems removed
- ¼ cup olive oil
- ¼ cup lemon juice

- ¼ cup coarsely chopped fresh basil
- Two cloves of garlic, peeled and minced

Directions:
- ➤ Combine the eggplant, red bell peppers, zucchini, and fresh mushrooms in a medium mixing dish.
- ➤ Combine the olive oil, lemon juice, basil, and garlic in a medium mixing bowl. Pour the mixture over the veggies, cover, and refrigerate for at least 1 hour.
- ➤ Preheat a high-heat outside grill.
- ➤ Place veggies on skewers or directly on the grill. Cook for 2 to 3 minutes per side on the preheated grill, coating regularly with the marinade, or until done to preference.

Quick Mediterranean Vegetables

Preparation Time: 10 minutes
Cooking Time: 15 minutes
Servings: 1

Ingredients:
- One tablespoon of olive oil
- ½ onion, chopped
- Two carrots, sliced
- One green bell pepper, cubed
- One red bell pepper, cubed
- One fennel bulb, thinly sliced
- Two teaspoons of dried Italian herb mix, or to taste
- salt and freshly ground black pepper to taste

Directions:
- ➤ Heat the olive oil and sauté the onion until tender and transparent in a large pan, about 5 minutes. Cook, occasionally turning, until carrots, bell peppers, and fennel are cooked but still firm to the bite, 5 to 10 minutes. Season with salt, pepper, and Italian herbs.

Hearty Turkey Stew with Vegetables

Preparation Time: 10 minutes
Cooking Time: 15 minutes
Servings: 1

Ingredients:
- Two tablespoons butter
- Two onions, chopped
- One stalk of celery, cut into 1-inch pieces
- Two carrots, peeled and sliced into 1-inch pieces
- Two potatoes, peeled and cubed
- Three tablespoons of all-purpose flour
- 3 cups chicken stock
- ¼ teaspoon dried marjoram
- Two skinless, boneless turkey breast halves, cubed
- One green bell pepper, diced

Directions:
- ➤ In a medium saucepan, melt the butter. Cook until the onions are soft in the pot. Cook until celery and carrots are soft. Combine the potatoes and flour in a mixing bowl. Season the soup with marjoram after adding the chicken stock. Bring the turkey to a boil in the pot. Reduce the heat to low, cover, and leave to simmer for 30 minutes.
- ➤ Cook for another 10 minutes, or until the green bell pepper is soft, in the soup.

Vegan Oven-Roasted Vegetables

Preparation Time: 10 minutes
Cooking Time: 15 minutes
Servings: 1

Ingredients:
- Six small red potatoes
- Four small leeks, chopped
- Four large carrots, peeled and cut into large chunks
- Two medium red onions, peeled and quartered
- Two red bell peppers, seeded and cut into wide strips
- ½ pound fresh shiitake mushroom stems removed
- One tablespoon olive oil, or more as needed
- ½ teaspoon thyme
- ¼ teaspoon salt
- ¼ teaspoon pepper

Directions:
- ➤ Fill a saucepan halfway with water to just below the bottom of the steamer insert. Bring a pot of water to a boil. Cover and cook the potatoes for 20 minutes or until tender. Drain thoroughly.
- ➤ Preheat the oven carefully to 400° F. (200 degrees C). Grease a 13x9-inch baking dish lightly.
- ➤ Cut each potato into 2 to 3 big slices and place them at the edges of the baking dish. Arrange leeks next to potatoes, then carrots, onions, red peppers, and mushrooms on top of and around the leeks and potatoes. Drizzle olive oil over veggies and season with thyme, salt, and pepper.
- ➤ Roast for 45 to 60 minutes, basting with pan juices every 15 minutes until veggies are soft when pierced with a fork.

One Pan Cheesy Chicken and Vegetables

Preparation Time: 10 minutes
Cooking Time: 15 minutes
Servings: 1

Ingredients:
- One tablespoon of olive oil
- 1 pound skinless, boneless chicken thighs, cut into strips
- One medium onion, finely diced
- Two medium carrots, peeled and diced
- Two stalks of celery, diced
- 1 (5.6 ounces) package Knorr® Rice Sides™ - Chicken
- 2 cups water
- 1 ½ teaspoon dried basil
- ¾ cup shredded Cheddar cheese

Directions:
- ➤ In a nonstick skillet, heat the oil over medium-high heat. Cook and stir the chicken until it is cooked through (no longer pink in the centre). Place the chicken in a bowl.
- ➤ Cook, stirring regularly, until the diced onion, carrot, and celery soften for about 5 minutes. Season with salt and pepper to taste. Stir in the Knorr® Rice Sides™ - Chicken flavour and water. Bring to a boil over high heat, then lower to medium-low and cover for 7 minutes.
- ➤ Combine cooked chicken, basil, and shredded Cheddar cheese in a mixing bowl.

Brian (Greek Mixed Vegetables in Tomato Sauce)

Preparation Time: 10 minutes
Cooking Time: 15 minutes
Servings: 1

Ingredients:
- Four tomatoes
- ½ cup olive oil
- Two tablespoons of red wine vinegar
- Two tablespoons of white sugar
- ⅓ cup chopped fresh parsley
- ⅓ cup chopped fresh mint
- ⅓ cup chopped fresh basil
- Two tablespoons of fresh oregano
- ¼ cup capers
- Two cloves garlic

- salt and ground black pepper to taste
- Two tablespoons of olive oil
- Two onions, sliced
- Two potatoes, sliced
- Two eggplants, sliced
- Three zucchini, sliced
- Three green bell peppers, sliced
- 2 cups okra

Directions:
- ➤ Preheat the oven carefully to 350°F (175 degrees C). In a food processor, combine three tomatoes, 1/2 cup olive oil, red wine vinegar, sugar, parsley, mint, basil, oregano, capers, and garlic to make a fresh tomato sauce. Set aside and season with salt and black pepper. Set aside the leftover tomato.
- ➤ In a pan over medium heat, heat the two tablespoons of olive oil and sauté and toss the onions until slightly brown, about 10 minutes.
- ➤ Combine the onions, potatoes, eggplant, zucchini, bell peppers, okra, the saved chopped tomato, and the fresh tomato sauce in a large baking dish. Add a little water to cover the veggies with sauce slightly.
- ➤ Bake in a preheated oven for 1 hour or until all veggies are soft.

Creole Vegetables

Preparation Time: 10 minutes
Cooking Time: 15 minutes
Servings: 1

Ingredients:
- ½ pound bacon
- Two tablespoons of bacon grease
- ½ cup finely chopped onion
- ½ cup finely chopped green bell pepper
- 2 cups chopped peeled tomatoes
- 2 cups chopped fresh green beans
- ¾ teaspoon salt
- ⅛ teaspoon pepper
- 1 ½ cups fresh corn kernels, cut from the cob
- Three tablespoons of all-purpose flour
- Three tablespoons water
- 1 cup evaporated milk

Directions:
- ➤ Cook bacon in a large pan over medium heat until uniformly browned. Set aside, leaving two tablespoons of bacon grease aside. In bacon grease, sauté the onion and green pepper until soft. Add tomatoes, green beans, salt, and pepper to taste. Simmer for 15 minutes, covered. Stir in the corn, cover, and simmer until the veggies are soft, approximately 20 minutes.
- ➤ Combine flour and water in a small mixing basin. Cook until the veggies are thickened, approximately 2 minutes. Remove from the heat and add the evaporated milk. Top with crumbled bacon. Serve right away.

Honey Curried Roasted Chicken and Vegetables

Preparation Time: 10 minutes
Cooking Time: 15 minutes
Servings: 1

Ingredients:
- 1 (3 pounds) whole chicken
- Four medium red potatoes, peeled and quartered
- Six carrots, cut into 1/2 inch pieces
- ⅔ cup honey
- ⅓ cup Dijon mustard
- Three tablespoons butter
- Two tablespoons of finely chopped onion

- 2 ½ teaspoons curry powder
- ½ teaspoon salt
- ¼ teaspoon red pepper flakes
- ¼ teaspoon ground ginger
- ¼ teaspoon finely chopped garlic
- 12 whole fresh mushrooms
- Two apples, cored and quartered (Optional)

Directions:
- ➤ Preheat the oven carefully to 350°F (175 degrees C).
- ➤ Roast the chicken breast side down in a roasting pan for 1 hour in a preheated oven.
- ➤ Bring the potatoes and carrots to a boil in a saucepan with enough water to cover—Cook for 20 minutes, or until the vegetables are soft.
- ➤ Combine the honey, mustard, butter, onion, curry powder, salt, cayenne pepper, ginger, and garlic. Bring to a boil while continually stirring. Set aside after removing from the heat.
- ➤ Remove the roasting pan drippings. Surround the chicken with potatoes, carrots, mushrooms, and apples. Drizzle the honey mixture over the chicken and veggies. Cook for another 20 minutes, or until the glaze has browned. The internal temperature of the chicken flesh should be 180 degrees F. (85 degrees C).

Broiled Portobello Mushrooms with Sauteed Vegetables

Preparation Time: 10 minutes
Cooking Time: 15 minutes
Servings: 1

Ingredients:
- ¼ cup balsamic vinegar
- ¼ cup olive oil
- Five sprigs of fresh thyme leave stripped
- One medium lemon, juiced
- Two large portobello mushroom caps
- salt and ground black pepper to taste
- Two tablespoons of olive oil
- One zucchini, chopped
- One red bell pepper, chopped
- One medium beefsteak tomato, diced
- Two-piece (blank)s artichoke hearts, drained and chopped
- Two cloves of garlic, minced
- Ten leaves of fresh basil, chopped
- ¼ cup panko bread crumbs
- ½ cup grated Parmesan cheese, divided

Directions:
- ➤ In a measuring cup, combine the balsamic vinegar, 14 cups of olive oil, and thyme. Pour the lemon juice into the marinade through a sieve (to keep the seeds out). The marinade should be whisked until the olive oil, and balsamic vinegar is evenly combined.
- ➤ Place the mushroom caps in a glass dish suitable for marinating. Pour over the balsamic marinade, cover, and set aside 15 minutes.
- ➤ Meanwhile, Preheat the oven carefully to 400°F (200 degrees C)—wrap foil around a metal baking dish.
- ➤ Transfer the mushrooms to the prepared baking dish, gills up, and season with salt and pepper.
- ➤ Bake for 30 minutes in a preheated oven.
- ➤ Heat two tablespoons of oil in a pan over medium heat while the mushrooms bake. For 10 minutes, sauté the zucchini and bell pepper in heated oil—Cook for 5 minutes after adding the tomato, artichoke hearts, garlic, and basil. Remove from the fire and stir in the panko bread crumbs and 1/4 cup Parmesan cheese.
- ➤ When the mushrooms are done baking, remove them from the oven and top with the sautéed mixture. Finish with the remaining Parmesan cheese. Turn on the broiler in the oven.

- ➤ Broil with the oven door open for 2 minutes, or until the Parmesan cheese on top is bubbling. Remove the skillet from the heat and, using a spatula, transfer the mushrooms to a serving platter with the sautéed veggies. Serve right away.

Roasted Indian-Spiced Vegetables

Preparation Time: 10 minutes
Cooking Time: 15 minutes
Servings: 1

Ingredients:
- Three tablespoons of olive oil
- Two teaspoons of garam masala
- One teaspoon salt
- Two medium potatoes, peeled and cut into 1-inch cubes
- 2 cups cauliflower florets
- One medium yellow onion, cut into 1/2-inch wedges
- Two tablespoons of minced cilantro

Directions:
- ➤ Preheat the oven carefully to 425° F. (220 degrees C). Using parchment paper, line a baking sheet.
- ➤ Combine the olive oil, garam masala, and salt in a small bowl. In a large mixing basin, combine the potatoes, cauliflower, and onion. Toss with the oil mixture to coat. Arrange the veggies on the prepared baking sheet.
- ➤ 30 to 35 minutes in a preheated oven, stirring every 10 minutes until veggies are soft and edges are browned. Remove from the oven and top with the cilantro.

Vegetable Dip

Preparation Time: 10 minutes
Cooking Time: 15 minutes
Servings: 1

Ingredients:
- ⅔ cup mayonnaise
- ⅔ cup sour cream
- 2 teaspoons Beau Monde ™ seasoning
- One tablespoon of dried dill weed
- One tablespoon of dried parsley
- One tablespoon of minced onion

Directions:
- ➤ Combine mayonnaise, sour cream, Beau Monde spice, dill, parsley, and chopped onion in a mixing bowl. Blend well. Refrigerate for at least four hours before serving.

Teriyaki Grilled Vegetables

Preparation Time: 10 minutes
Cooking Time: 15 minutes
Servings: 1

Ingredients:
- 8 ounces portobello mushrooms, cleaned and stems cut
- One yellow onion, cut into wedges
- One zucchini, cut into 1/4-inch diagonal slices
- One yellow squash, sliced diagonally into 1/2-inch pieces
- One yellow bell pepper, cut into 1-inch pieces
- One orange bell pepper, cut into 1-inch pieces
- ⅓ cup teriyaki baste and glaze
- One clove of minced garlic
- ¼ teaspoon ground black pepper

Directions:
- ➤ Preheat an outside grill over medium-high heat and grease the grate liberally.
- ➤ In a large mixing basin, combine the mushrooms, onion, zucchini, yellow squash, and bell peppers. Mix in the teriyaki sauce, garlic, and ground pepper. Toss to cover the veggies completely with the sauce; be careful with the onion to keep it intact.

➤ Place the veggies on the grill and cook, rotating once, for 5 to 10 minutes, or until they begin to soften.

Grilled Vegetables with Homemade Teriyaki Sauce

Preparation Time: 10 minutes
Cooking Time: 15 minutes
Servings: 1

Ingredients:
- 2 cups fresh broccoli florets
- Ten baby carrots halved lengthwise
- Four-button mushrooms, sliced
- One small zucchini, sliced into rounds
- One tablespoon of olive oil
- Teriyaki Sauce:
- ½ cup soy sauce
- ½ cup white sugar
- ¼ cup apple cider vinegar
- One tablespoon of toasted sesame seeds
- One tablespoon cornstarch
- Two teaspoons of garlic powder
- One teaspoon of ginger paste

Directions:
➤ Preheat an outside grill over medium-high heat and grease the grate liberally. Preheat the grill's side burner to medium heat.
➤ Combine the broccoli, carrots, mushrooms, and zucchini in a large mixing basin. Drizzle with olive oil and toss to coat. Fill a grill basket halfway with veggies.
➤ Stir the soy sauce, sugar, vinegar, sesame seeds, cornstarch, garlic powder, and ginger paste in a medium saucepan. Place the saucepan on the grill's side burner and cook until it begins to boil, about 5 minutes; lower heat to low and simmer.
➤ While the sauce cooks, grill the veggies for 15 minutes, turning every 5 minutes. Pour the teriyaki sauce over the veggies and toss to incorporate. Cook for another 5 minutes, or until the vegetables are soft.

Baked Vegetables I

Preparation Time: 10 minutes
Cooking Time: 15 minutes
Servings: 1

Ingredients:
- Two potatoes, peeled and cubed
- Four carrots, cut into 1-inch pieces
- One head of fresh broccoli, cut into florets
- Four zucchini, thickly sliced
- salt to taste
- ¼ cup olive oil
- 1 (1 ounce) package of dry onion soup mix

Directions:
➤ Preheat the oven carefully to 400°F (200 degrees C). Grease a big, shallow baking dish lightly.
➤ Place the veggies in the prepared baking dish and season gently. Brush with olive oil, then top with dry soup mix.
➤ Bake for 30 to 45 minutes, or until veggies are soft, in a preheated oven. When they are done, you may test them with a fork.

Stir-Fried Vegetables

Preparation Time: 10 minutes
Cooking Time: 15 minutes
Servings: 1

Ingredients:
- Two tablespoons of light soy sauce
- One teaspoon of ground ginger
- Two tablespoons of all-purpose flour

- 1 cup low-sodium chicken broth
- ¼ cup cold water
- Three tablespoons of vegetable oil
- Four green bell peppers, cut into matchsticks
- Four carrots, cut into matchsticks
- 2 cups broccoli florets
- Eight mushrooms, sliced

Directions:
➤ In a small bowl, combine the soy sauce and ginger. Combine the flour, chicken broth, and water in a separate basin.
➤ Cook and stir peppers, carrots, broccoli, and mushrooms in a large pan or wok over high heat until barely tender, approximately 3 minutes.
➤ Cook and stir for 1 minute after tossing veggies with soy sauce mixture. Stir the flour mixture into the veggies gradually; bring to a boil and simmer until thickened, approximately 3 minutes.

Vegetarian Meatloaf with Vegetables

Preparation Time: 10 minutes
Cooking Time: 15 minutes
Servings: 1

Ingredients:
- ½ (14 ounces) package of vegetarian ground beef (e.g., Gimme Lean TM)
- 1 (12 ounces) package of vegetarian burger crumbles
- One onion, chopped
- Two eggs, beaten
- Two tablespoons of vegetarian Worcestershire sauce
- One teaspoon salt
- ⅓ teaspoon pepper
- One teaspoon of ground sage
- ½ teaspoon garlic powder
- Two teaspoons of prepared mustard
- One tablespoon of vegetable oil
- 3 ½ slices bread, cubed
- ⅓ cup milk
- 1 (8 ounces) can of tomato sauce
- Four carrots, cut into 1-inch pieces
- Four potatoes, cubed
- One cooking spray

Directions:
➤ Preheat the oven carefully to 350°F (175 degrees C).
➤ Combine vegetarian ground beef, crumbled vegetarian ground beef, onion, eggs, Worcestershire sauce, salt, pepper, sage, garlic powder, mustard, oil, bread cubes, and milk in a large mixing bowl. Form the mixture into a loaf in a 9 x 13-inch baking dish. Top with tomato sauce.
➤ Spray the carrots and potatoes around the loaf with cooking spray.
➤ Bake for 30 to 45 minutes, turning veggies halfway through. Bake for a further 30 to 45 minutes. Allow standing for 15 minutes before slicing.

Vegetable Whip

Preparation Time: 10 minutes
Cooking Time: 15 minutes
Servings: 1

Ingredients:
- One turnip, peeled and diced
- Four carrots - peeled and diced
- One large onion, chopped
- Six medium potatoes - peeled and cubed
- ¼ cup butter
- ½ cup milk
- salt and pepper to taste

Directions:

- Cover the turnip, carrots, onion, and potatoes with water in a saucepan. Bring to a boil over medium-high heat and simmer until the potatoes are fork-tender.
- Drain the veggies and toss in the butter until it has melted. Using an electric mixer, beat till light and fluffy, gradually adding milk. Beat for a short time, just until smooth. Season with salt and pepper to taste, and serve immediately.

Chicken and Vegetables Soup

Preparation Time: 10 minutes
Cooking Time: 15 minutes
Servings: 1

Ingredients:
- One whole onion, peeled
- Six chicken drumsticks
- ½ teaspoon salt
- ⅓ head cauliflower, chopped
- 1 pound Brussels sprouts, trimmed and chopped
- ½ pound baby carrots, chopped
- 1 pound fresh asparagus spears, trimmed and chopped
- 1 (32 ounces) package of fat-free chicken broth
- ½ teaspoon garlic powder
- One teaspoon salt-free seasoning blend
- ¼ cup uncooked long-grain white rice
- One bunch of fresh dill weed

Directions:
- Fill a saucepan halfway with cold water and add the onion and chicken. Bring to a boil, season with salt, and serve. Cook for 30 minutes, or until the chicken flesh comes easily off the bone. Remove the chicken from the pot, leaving the water behind. Remove the onion. Remove all flesh off the bones, cut it, and return it to the saucepan. Remove the bones.
- Combine the cauliflower, Brussels sprouts, tiny carrots, and asparagus in the pot. Add the chicken broth—season with garlic powder and a salt-free spice mix to taste. Bring to a boil, lower to low heat and cook for 40 minutes.
- Incorporate the rice into the saucepan. Cook for another 20 minutes, or until the rice is soft. Five minutes before serving, stir in the dill.

CHAPTER 17: VEGAN

Vegan Zucchini Brownies

Preparation Time: 10 minutes
Cooking Time: 15 minutes
Servings: 1

Ingredients:
- cooking spray
- 1 cup white sugar
- ½ cup brown sugar
- ½ cup olive oil
- One tablespoon of vanilla extract
- 2 cups all-purpose flour
- ½ cup cocoa powder (such as Hershey's®)
- 1 ½ teaspoons baking soda
- One teaspoon salt
- 3 cups shredded zucchini
- 1 cup vegan chocolate chips

Directions:
- Preheat the oven carefully to 350° F. (175 degrees C). Coat a 9-inch square baking pan with cooking spray.
- In a large mixing basin, add the sugar, brown sugar, and olive oil; beat with an electric mixer until thoroughly blended. Blend in the vanilla extract. Mix the flour, cocoa powder, baking soda, and salt until well blended. (The mixture will be dry.)
- Mix in the zucchini with a spoon until well combined. Allow for 5 minutes to allow the mixture to become moister. Mix in the vegan chocolate chips. Pour the batter into the prepared pan.
- Bake for 25 to 30 minutes, or until the top is dry and the edges begin to come away from the sides of the pan. Allow cooling fully before cutting.

Vegan Mug Brownie

Preparation Time: 10 minutes
Cooking Time: 15 minutes
Servings: 1

Ingredients:
- ¼ cup whole wheat flour
- Two teaspoons of white sugar, or to taste
- Two teaspoons of unsweetened cocoa powder
- ¼ teaspoon baking soda
- One pinch salt
- ¼ cup water
- Two tablespoons of canola oil
- ⅛ teaspoon vanilla extract
- Two teaspoons of vegan chocolate chips (such as Enjoy Life®)

Directions:
- Combine whole wheat flour, white sugar, cocoa powder, baking soda, and salt in a microwave-safe cup. Incorporate the water, canola oil, and vanilla extract. Stir in the chocolate chunks.
- Microwave for 50 seconds to 1 minute, or until thoroughly cooked.

Vegan Lasagna I

Preparation Time: 10 minutes
Cooking Time: 15 minutes
Servings: 1

Ingredients:
- Two tablespoons of olive oil
- 1 ½ cup chopped onion
- Three tablespoons of minced garlic
- 4 (14.5 ounces) cans of stewed tomatoes
- ⅓ cup tomato paste
- ½ cup chopped fresh basil
- ½ cup chopped parsley
- One teaspoon salt
- One teaspoon of ground black pepper
- 1 (16 ounces) package of lasagna noodles
- 2 pounds firm tofu
- Two tablespoons of minced garlic
- ¼ cup chopped fresh basil
- ¼ cup chopped parsley
- ½ teaspoon salt
- ground black pepper to taste
- 3 (10 ounces) packages frozen chopped spinach, thawed and drained

Directions:
- Heat the olive oil in a big, heavy saucepan over medium heat to make the sauce. Sauté the onions in the pot for 5 minutes, or until they are tender. Cook for 5 minutes more after adding the garlic.
- Combine the tomatoes, tomato paste, basil, and parsley in a saucepan. Stir thoroughly, reduce the heat to low, and cover the sauce for 1 hour—season with salt and pepper.
- Bring a big pot of salted water to a boil while the sauce is simmering. Boil the lasagna noodles for 9 minutes before draining and rinsing well.
- Preheat the oven carefully to 400° F. (200 degrees C).
- In a large mixing basin, combine the tofu blocks. Combine the garlic, basil, and parsley in a mixing bowl. Add the salt and pepper, then mash everything together by squeezing tofu chunks with your fingers. Combine thoroughly.
- Make the lasagna: 1 cup tomato sauce, spread in the bottom of a 9x13 inch casserole pan. Arrange a single layer of lasagna noodles, then top with one-third of the tofu mixture. Spread the spinach equally on top of the tofu. Next, spoon 1 1/2 cups of tomato sauce over the tofu, followed by another layer of noodles. Then, sprinkle another third of the tofu mixture over the noodles, cover with 1 1/2 cups tomato sauce, and finish with a final layer of noodles on top of the tomato sauce. Finally, distribute the remaining tomato sauce over the noodles and top with 1/3 of the tofu.
- Bake the lasagna for 30 minutes, covered in foil. Serve immediately and enjoy.

Vegan Mug Cake

Preparation Time: 10 minutes
Cooking Time: 15 minutes
Servings: 1

Ingredients:
- Four tablespoons of all-purpose flour
- Three tablespoons of white sugar
- Two tablespoons of unsweetened cocoa powder
- ¼ teaspoon baking powder
- Four tablespoons applesauce
- Three tablespoons of soy milk
- One tablespoon of vegan chocolate chips, or more to taste
- One tablespoon of toasted flaked coconut (Optional)

Directions:
- Combine the flour, sugar, cocoa powder, and baking powder in a cup. Combine applesauce and soy milk in a separate dish, then add to the flour mixture. Stir until well

blended. Fold in the chocolate chips and top with the coconut.

- ➢ Microwave on high for 3 minutes, or until the mug cake has set and risen nicely.

Vegan Banh Mi

Preparation Time: 10 minutes
Cooking Time: 15 minutes
Servings: 1

Ingredients:

- ½ cup vegan Worcestershire sauce
- ½ cup tamari soy sauce
- ½ cup water
- One shiitake mushroom
- One tablespoon of fermented black bean paste
- One tablespoon of minced shallot
- One clove of garlic, crushed
- One strip of nori seaweed
- 4 ½ ounces tempeh
- ¼ cup vegan mayonnaise
- One teaspoon of sriracha sauce
- 1 (6 inches) French baguette, sliced into bite-sized cubes
- One tablespoon of olive oil
- One jalapeno pepper, sliced
- ½ ounce pickled daikon, or to taste
- ½ ounce pickled carrot, or to taste
- Two cucumber slices, or to taste
- Three tablespoons of chopped fresh cilantro

Directions:

- ➢ Preheat the oven carefully to 350° F. (175 degrees C). Using parchment paper, line a baking sheet.
- ➢ In a saucepan over medium heat, combine Worcestershire sauce, tamari, water, mushroom, black bean paste, shallot, garlic clove, and seaweed. Remove from the heat and set aside to cool. Remove the sauce from the heat and discard the solids.
- ➢ Pour 1/3 cup of the sauce over the tempeh in a bowl. Marinate for 20 minutes, rotating tempeh halfway through.
- ➢ Mix one teaspoon of the tempeh marinade, vegan mayo, and sriracha in a separate dish. Refrigerate until ready to use.
- ➢ Arrange the baguette slices on the prepared baking sheet and sprinkle olive oil. Toss the bread and place it in a single layer.
- ➢ Bake for 15 minutes in a preheated oven. Cook until the bread is browned, approximately 8 minutes more. Transfer to a mixing basin.
- ➢ Place the tempeh on a baking sheet and set aside the liquid. Bake for 10 minutes, basting halfway with some of the remaining marinade. Bake for 10 minutes more, basting halfway through.
- ➢ Tempeh should be cut into cubes. Fill serving dishes with bread, tempeh, jalapeño pieces, pickled daikon, carrot, cucumber, and cilantro. Serve with sriracha mayo on top.

Vegan Almond Paste

Preparation Time: 10 minutes
Cooking Time: 15 minutes
Servings: 1

Ingredients:

- 1 cup blanched whole almonds
- ½ cup white sugar
- One tablespoon of white sugar
- ¼ cup water
- ⅛ teaspoon almond extract

Directions:

- ➢ In a food processor, pulse almonds to a meal-like consistency, scraping down the sides and the bottom of the

bowl as needed. Don't overprocess it; the mixture should still be crumbly, not paste-like, at this point.

- ➢ Combine 1/2 cup plus one tablespoon of sugar and water in a small saucepan. Bring to a boil and simmer for 4 minutes over medium heat. Continue to heat until it hits 240 degrees F (115 degrees C) and is a medium-thick syrup, about 6 to 8 minutes longer. If you overcook the syrup, it will solidify as it cools.
- ➢ Take the pan off the heat and mix in the almonds and almond essence. Return to the heat and cook, stirring with a spatula and scraping over the bottom and along the sides of the pan to prevent burning, for 30 to 60 seconds, or until the almond paste holds together. Cooking it for too long will cause it to caramelize.
- ➢ Take the pan off the heat. When cool enough to handle, use immediately, or wrap in waxed paper and preserve in an airtight container for up to a few weeks. Alternatively, place the wrapped almond paste in a freezer bag and store it in the freezer for up to six months.

Vegan Basic Vanilla Cake

Preparation Time: 10 minutes
Cooking Time: 15 minutes
Servings: 1

Ingredients:

- 1 cup plain soy milk
- One tablespoon of apple cider vinegar
- 1 ½ cups unbleached all-purpose flour
- 1 cup white sugar
- One teaspoon of baking soda
- One teaspoon of baking powder
- ½ teaspoon salt
- ⅓ cup canola oil
- ¼ cup water
- One tablespoon of lemon juice
- One tablespoon of vanilla extract
- ¼ teaspoon almond extract

Directions:

- ➢ Preheat the oven carefully to 350°F (175 degrees C). 8x8-inch baking dish, greased and floured
- ➢ In a large glass measuring cup, combine the soy milk and vinegar.
- ➢ Combine the flour, sugar, baking soda, baking powder, and salt in a mixing dish.
- ➢ Quickly combine canola oil, water, lemon juice, vanilla extract, and almond extract into the soy milk mixture using a fork. Stir in the soy milk mixture until the batter is lump-free. Pour the batter into the baking dish that has been prepared.
- ➢ Bake for 35 minutes, or until a toothpick inserted into the middle of the cake comes out clean.

Mushroom Stroganoff (Vegan)

Preparation Time: 10 minutes
Cooking Time: 15 minutes
Servings: 1

Ingredients:

- 8 ounces oyster mushrooms
- One tablespoon oil, or to taste
- One small onion, diced
- One tablespoon of all-purpose flour
- 1 cup almond milk
- One tablespoon of lemon juice
- salt and ground black pepper to taste

Directions:

- ➢ With a fork, shred the mushrooms.
- ➢ In a skillet over medium-high heat, heat the oil. Fry the mushrooms and onion for 2 to 3 minutes, or until tender. Stir in the flour and cook for another minute.

> Combine almond milk and lemon juice in a mixing bowl. Cook for 7 to 8 minutes. Season with salt and pepper to taste.

Vegan Stuffing

Preparation Time: 10 minutes
Cooking Time: 15 minutes
Servings: 1

Ingredients:

- One loaf of vegan, gluten-free, brown rice bread (such as Food for Life®), cubed
- Two tablespoons of vegan margarine (such as Earth Balance®)
- 1 ½ cups mixed forest mushrooms, diced
- One ¼ cup sweet onion, chopped
- 2 ½ teaspoons dried sage
- 1 ½ teaspoon dried rosemary
- ½ teaspoon dried thyme
- sea salt and freshly ground black pepper to taste
- Six tablespoons of vegan margarine (such as Earth Balance®), melted
- 1 ½ cups low-sodium vegan broth
- 8 ounces fresh cranberries
- 1 cup Granny Smith apple, peeled and chopped
- ⅓ cup minced fresh parsley

Directions:

> Preheat the oven carefully to 350° F. (175 degrees C). Aluminium foil should be used to line a baking pan.
> Place the bread cubes on the baking sheet that has been prepared. Toast for 10 minutes in a preheated oven until aromatic and slightly brown. Remove from the oven, but leave the oven on. Allow the bread to cool before transferring it to a large mixing dish.
> While the bread is toasting, melt two tablespoons of margarine in a large saucepan over medium heat. Mix in the mushrooms and onions. Cook for 5 minutes, or until the onions are slightly transparent. If more moisture is required, add a dash of vegetable broth—season with sage, rosemary, thyme, salt, and black pepper to taste. Cook and whisk with a wooden spoon for another 2 minutes or until blended.
> Combine the mushroom mixture and the toasted bread in a mixing basin. Toss to distribute evenly. Pour six tablespoons of melted margarine and vegan broth over the mixture—mix in the cranberries, apple, and parsley. Thoroughly but gently combine. Cover the stuffing in a casserole dish with aluminium wrap.
> Bake for 45 minutes in a preheated oven; check at 25 minutes to prevent burning. Uncover and gently stir. Bake for another 15 minutes, or until the top is golden. Allow it cool for a few minutes before serving.

Vegan Baked Oatmeal Patties

Preparation Time: 10 minutes
Cooking Time: 15 minutes
Servings: 1

Ingredients:

- 4 cups water
- 4 cups quick-cooking oats
- ½ onion, chopped
- ⅓ cup vegetable oil
- ½ cup spaghetti sauce
- ½ cup chopped pecans
- ¼ cup nutritional yeast
- Two teaspoons of garlic powder
- One teaspoon of dried basil
- Two teaspoons of onion powder
- One teaspoon of ground coriander
- One teaspoon sage

- One teaspoon of active dry yeast

Directions:

> Preheat the oven carefully to 350°F (175 degrees C). A baking sheet should be greased.
> Bring the water to a boil, then add the oatmeal. Reduce the heat to low and cover. Cook for 5 to 10 minutes, or until the oats are tender and the liquid has been absorbed. Remove from the heat and set aside for 5 minutes.
> Add the onion, oil, spaghetti sauce, pecans, nutritional yeast, garlic powder, basil, onion powder, coriander, sage, and active yeast to the oats. Form into patties after thoroughly mixing. Place on a baking sheet that has been prepared.
Fifteen minutes in the oven. Bake for another 15 minutes on the other side.

Vegan Potatoes au Gratin

Preparation Time: 10 minutes
Cooking Time: 15 minutes
Servings: 1

Ingredients:

- Six large potatoes, peeled and cubed
- One ¼ cups vegetable broth, divided
- Two tablespoons of all-purpose flour
- One teaspoon of seasoning salt
- ½ teaspoon ground black pepper
- ¼ teaspoon dry mustard
- ⅛ teaspoon nutmeg
- 2 cups soy milk
- 1 ½ cups shredded Cheddar-flavored soy cheese, divided
- 1 cup soft bread crumbs
- Three teaspoons paprika

Directions:

> Preheat the oven carefully to 350 degrees F (175 degrees C).
> Bring a large pot of salted water to a boil. Add potatoes and cook until tender but still firm, about 15 minutes. Drain and place in a 9 x 13-inch baking dish.
> Meanwhile, boil two tablespoons of broth in a small saucepan over high heat. Reduce heat to low. Stir in flour, seasoning salt, pepper, mustard and nutmeg. Gradually add soy milk, constantly stirring until thickened. Stir in half of the soy cheese. Stir constantly until the cheese is melted. Pour over potatoes.
> In a small bowl, combine the remaining broth and the bread crumbs. Spoon evenly over potatoes. Top with remaining soy cheese. Sprinkle with paprika.
> Bake in preheated oven for 20 minutes.

Vegan Pancakes

Preparation Time: 10 minutes
Cooking Time: 15 minutes
Servings: 1

Ingredients:

- One ¼ cup all-purpose flour
- Two tablespoons of white sugar
- Two teaspoons of baking powder
- ½ teaspoon salt
- One ¼ cup of water
- One tablespoon oil

Directions:

> In a large mixing basin, sift together the flour, sugar, baking powder, and salt; form a well in the middle. In a separate bowl, whisk together the water and oil; pour into the flour mixture. Stir only until combined; the mixture will be lumpy.
> Over medium-high heat, heat a lightly greased griddle.
> Drop batter onto the griddle in big spoonfuls. Cook until bubbles appear and the edges are dry. Cook until the bottoms are browned, 1 to 2 minutes. Rep with the remaining batter.

Vegan Irish Stew

Preparation Time: 10 minutes
Cooking Time: 15 minutes
Servings: 1

Ingredients:
- ¼ cup extra-virgin olive oil
- Three leeks, thinly sliced
- 1 cup chopped red potatoes
- 1 cup peeled and sliced parsnips
- 1 cup peeled and chopped turnip
- 1 cup sliced celery
- 1 cup sliced carrots
- 4 cups garbanzo beans, drained
- 4 cups low-sodium vegetable broth
- 2 cups vegan stout beer (such as Samuel Smith's)
- ½ cup chopped fresh parsley
- ¼ teaspoon dried rosemary
- ¼ teaspoon dried thyme
- ¼ teaspoon dried marjoram
- ¼ cup water (Optional)
- salt and ground black pepper to taste

Directions:
- ➢ In a large saucepan, heat the olive oil over medium-high heat. Cook until the leeks are transparent, 3 to 5 minutes. Potatoes, parsnips, turnips, celery, and carrots should be added—Cook and stir for 4 minutes, or until somewhat soft and covered with oil. Garbanzo beans, vegetable broth, beer, and parsley are all optional. Heat the stew to a boil.
- ➢ Cook until the veggies are soft and the stew has thickened somewhat, approximately 1 hour more. If required, add a splash of water—season with salt and pepper to taste.

Simple Vegan Coleslaw

Preparation Time: 10 minutes
Cooking Time: 15 minutes
Servings: 1

Ingredients:
- 1 (16 ounces) bag coleslaw mix
- ⅔ cup vegan mayonnaise (such as Follow Your Heart® Vegenaise®)
- ½ cup granular sucralose sweetener (such as Splenda®)
- Three tablespoons of olive oil
- One tablespoon of white vinegar
- One tablespoon of poppy seeds
- ¼ teaspoon salt

Directions:
- ➢ In a large mixing bowl, combine the coleslaw ingredients. Combine vegan mayonnaise, sweetener, olive oil, vinegar, poppy seeds, and salt in a small mixing dish. Slowly fold the dressing into the coleslaw mixture.
- ➢ Before serving, chill the coleslaw for at least 2 hours. Serve chilled.

Vegan Mac and No Cheese

Preparation Time: 10 minutes
Cooking Time: 15 minutes
Servings: 1

Ingredients:
- 1 (8 ounces) package of uncooked elbow macaroni
- One tablespoon of vegetable oil
- One medium onion, chopped
- 1 cup cashews
- ⅓ cup lemon juice
- One ⅓ cup of water
- salt to taste
- ⅓ cup canola oil
- 4 ounces roasted red peppers, drained

- Three tablespoons of nutritional yeast
- One teaspoon of garlic powder
- One teaspoon of onion powder

Directions:
- ➢ Preheat the oven carefully to 350°F (175 degrees C).
- ➢ Warm up a big saucepan of gently salted water. Cook for 8 to 10 minutes, or until the macaroni is al dente; drain. Place in a medium baking dish.
- ➢ In a medium saucepan over medium heat, heat the vegetable oil. Cook until the onion is soft and gently browned. Gently fold in the macaroni.
- ➢ Cashews, lemon juice, water, and salt should be combined in a blender or food processor. Blend gradually in the canola oil, roasted red peppers, nutritional yeast, garlic powder, and onion powder. Blend until completely smooth. Mix in the pasta and onions well.
- ➢ Bake for 45 minutes, or until gently browned, in a preheated oven. Allow 10 to 15 minutes to cool before serving.

Vegan Jalapeno Poppers

Preparation Time: 10 minutes
Cooking Time: 15 minutes
Servings: 1

Ingredients:
- 12 medium jalapeno peppers, sliced in half and seeded
- One tablespoon of vegetable oil
- 1 (8 ounces) package of button mushrooms, finely diced
- ½ cup finely diced onion
- Two cloves of garlic, minced
- 1 (8 ounces) tub vegan cream cheese substitute, softened
- 1 cup vegan shredded cheese substitute, divided
- salt and ground black pepper to taste

Directions:
- ➢ Preheat the oven carefully to 375° F. (190 degrees C). Place the jalapeno halves, open side up, on a baking sheet coated with aluminium foil.
- ➢ In a pan over medium-high heat, heat the vegetable oil. Sauté the mushrooms, onion, and garlic in the pan for 8 minutes, or until the veggies are soft and the mushrooms have shed their liquid. Transfer the veggies to a dish lined with paper towels to absorb any extra liquid.
- ➢ Combine the mushroom mixture, cream cheese substitute, 3/4 cup shredded cheese substitute, salt, and pepper in a mixing dish. Spoon into the halves of jalapeno peppers on the baking sheet.
- ➢ Bake for 20 minutes in a preheated oven.
- ➢ Remove from the oven and sprinkle the remaining 1/4 cup shredded cheese substitute on top. Broil for 1 to 2 minutes, or until the cheese is melted and slightly browned.

Vegan Jalapeno Cornbread in the Air Fryer

Preparation Time: 10 minutes
Cooking Time: 15 minutes
Servings: 1

Ingredients:
- One tablespoon of flaxseed meal
- Three tablespoons water
- cooking spray
- 1 cup stone-ground yellow cornmeal
- ⅔ cup all-purpose flour
- ¼ cup nutritional yeast
- Two tablespoons of white sugar
- Two ¼ teaspoons of baking powder
- One teaspoon of kosher salt
- ½ teaspoon ground black pepper
- 1 cup unsweetened almond milk
- ⅓ cup vegetable oil

- One large jalapeno pepper, seeded and minced, or to taste

Directions:
- ➢ Combine water and flaxseed meal in a small dish and set aside 10 minutes.
- ➢ Meanwhile, prepare an air fryer to 350°F (175°C) according to the manufacturer's directions. Coat a 6-inch heat-resistant inner pot with cooking spray.
- ➢ Combine cornmeal, flour, nutritional yeast, sugar, baking powder, salt, and pepper in a medium mixing bowl. Stir in the flaxseed and water combination, almond milk, and oil until just combined, and no lumps remain. Pour the prepared pot into the air fryer and stir in the jalapeño.
- ➢ Cook for 15 minutes in a preheated air fryer. Remove the inner pot with tongs, turn the cornbread, and continue to air fry for another 5 minutes, or until a toothpick inserted into the middle comes out clean. Serve hot.

Vegan Blueberry Muffins with Applesauce
Preparation Time: 10 minutes
Cooking Time: 15 minutes
Servings: 1

Ingredients:
- One cooking spray
- 2 cups fresh blueberries
- 2 cups all-purpose flour
- 1 cup lightly packed brown sugar
- ½ cup unsweetened applesauce
- ½ cup soy milk
- ¼ cup soy margarine
- One tablespoon of baking powder
- One teaspoon of vanilla extract
- ½ teaspoon salt

Directions:
- ➢ Preheat the oven carefully to 350° F. (175 degrees C). 12 tiny muffin cups lined with paper liners or sprayed with cooking spray
- ➢ Combine blueberries, flour, sugar, applesauce, soy milk, soy margarine, baking powder, vanilla extract, and salt in a mixing dish. Fill muffin cups 3/4 of the way with batter.
- ➢ Bake for 35 minutes in a preheated oven until the tops are crisp. Allow cooling gently on a rack.

Orange Vegan Cake
Preparation Time: 10 minutes
Cooking Time: 15 minutes
Servings: 1

Ingredients:

- One large orange, peeled
- 1 ½ cups all-purpose flour
- 1 cup white sugar
- ½ cup vegetable oil
- 1 ½ teaspoons baking soda
- ¼ teaspoon salt

Directions:
- ➢ Preheat the oven carefully to 375°F (190 degrees C). Grease an 8x8 baking dish.
- ➢ Blend the orange until it is liquified; measure 1 cup of orange juice.
- ➢ Combine orange juice, flour, sugar, vegetable oil, baking soda, and salt in a mixing dish. Pour the batter into the prepared baking dish.
- ➢ Bake for 30 minutes, or until a toothpick inserted into the middle of the cake comes out clean.

Easy Vegan Gingerbread Cookies
Preparation Time: 10 minutes
Cooking Time: 15 minutes
Servings: 1

Ingredients:
- 1 ½ cups all-purpose flour
- One teaspoon of baking powder
- One teaspoon of ground cinnamon
- ½ teaspoon baking soda
- ½ teaspoon ground ginger
- ½ teaspoon ground allspice
- ¼ teaspoon salt
- ½ cup coconut oil, at room temperature
- ⅓ cup molasses
- ¼ cup white sugar
- One teaspoon of vanilla extract

Directions:
- ➢ Preheat the oven carefully to 350°F (175 degrees C). 2 baking pans lined with parchment paper
- ➢ Combine the flour, baking powder, cinnamon, baking soda, ginger, allspice, and salt in a mixing bowl.
- ➢ Combine the coconut oil, molasses, and sugar; add the vanilla essence. Mix in the flour mixture for approximately 2 minutes or until a sticky dough forms. Wrap the dough in plastic wrap and place it in the refrigerator for 2 hours.
- ➢ Roll out the dough to a thickness of 1/4 to 1/2 inch on a floured surface. Flour the cookie cutter, cut out cookies and lay them on the prepared baking pans.
- ➢ 8 to 10 minutes in a preheated oven until gently browned.

CHAPTER 18: SALADS & SIDES

Christmas Pomegranate Salad

Preparation Time: 10 minutes
Cooking Time: 15 minutes
Servings: 1

Ingredients:
- 3 cups leafy salad green mix
- ½ cup pomegranate seeds
- ⅓ cup crumbled blue cheese
- ¼ cup crushed walnuts
- ¼ cup cranberry vinaigrette

Directions:
- ➤ In a medium-sized salad dish, combine leafy greens, pomegranate seeds, blue cheese, and walnuts. Just before serving, drizzle with cranberry vinaigrette.

Grilled Asparagus Salad

Preparation Time: 10 minutes
Cooking Time: 15 minutes
Servings: 1

Ingredients:
- ¼ cup olive oil
- ⅛ cup lemon juice
- 12 fresh asparagus spears
- 6 cups fresh spinach leaves
- ⅛ cup grated Parmesan cheese
- One tablespoon of seasoned slivered almonds

Directions:
- ➤ Preheat a grill to medium-low heat. On a dish, combine the lemon juice and olive oil. Roll the asparagus around on the platter to coat.
- ➤ Grill the asparagus for 5 minutes, flipping once and brushing with the olive oil mixture. Remove off the grill and return to the oil-covered plate.
- ➤ Combine the spinach, Parmesan cheese, and slivered almonds in a large mixing basin. Cut the asparagus into bite-size pieces and toss it into the salad with the lemon juice and oil from the dish. Toss to combine, then serve.

Marinated Carrot Salad

Preparation Time: 10 minutes
Cooking Time: 15 minutes
Servings: 1

Ingredients:
- 2 pounds carrots, sliced
- 1 (10.75 ounces) can of condensed tomato soup
- ¼ cup white sugar
- ½ cup white vinegar
- ¼ cup canola oil
- One teaspoon of prepared mustard
- One teaspoon of Worcestershire sauce
- ½ cup chopped celery
- ½ cup chopped green onion
- One green bell pepper, seeded and cut into strips

Directions:
- ➤ Bring a large saucepan of water to a boil, add the carrots and cook until soft, about 3 to 5 minutes. Set aside after draining.
- ➤ Whisk the soup, sugar, vinegar, oil, mustard, and Worcestershire sauce in a large mixing basin. Toss in the carrots, celery, onion, and pepper to coat. Refrigerate for at least 4 hours to enable the carrots to marinade.

Mexican Fiesta Pasta Salad

Preparation Time: 10 minutes
Cooking Time: 15 minutes
Servings: 1

Ingredients:
- 1 (16 ounces) package of dried rotini pasta
- 1 ½ cups medium chunky salsa
- 1 cup mayonnaise
- ½ cup sour cream
- 1 (16 ounces) can of black beans, rinsed and drained
- 1 (11 ounces) can of Mexican-style corn with red and green peppers, drained
- ½ cup chopped red bell pepper
- Two green onions, sliced thin
- 1 (4.25 ounce) can slice black olives, drained
- ½ teaspoon garlic powder
- ½ teaspoon ground cumin, or to taste
- ½ teaspoon dried cilantro, or to taste
- One teaspoon salt
- ground black pepper to taste

Directions:
- ➤ Bring a large saucepan of lightly salted water to a boil; cook the rotini in the boiling water for 8 minutes, or until the pasta is cooked through but firm to the biting. Drain. Rinse thoroughly under cold running water until totally cool.
- ➤ In a large mixing bowl, combine the salsa, mayonnaise, sour cream, black beans, Mexican-style corn, red bell pepper, green onions, black olives, garlic powder, cumin, cilantro, salt, and pepper; add the chilled pasta and toss to coat evenly. Refrigerate the bowl for 2 hours to overnight before serving, covered with plastic wrap.

Pasta Salad with Crab

Preparation Time: 10 minutes
Cooking Time: 15 minutes
Servings: 1

Ingredients:
- 1 pound uncooked tri-colour rotini pasta
- One tablespoon extra-virgin olive oil
- One green bell pepper, seeded and diced
- 2 cups broccoli florets
- 1 cup diced carrots
- 8 ounces fresh crabmeat, well picked over
- 2 ounces sliced black olives, drained
- Three tablespoons minced sweet onion
- 1 cup mayonnaise
- Six tablespoons of balsamic vinaigrette salad dressing
- One teaspoon of dried Italian herb seasoning
- ⅛ teaspoon ground black pepper, or to taste
- ¼ cup cherry tomatoes for garnish

Directions:
- ➤ Bring a large saucepan of lightly salted water to a boil; cook rotini for 8 minutes, or until cooked but firm to the biting. Drain pasta and toss with extra-virgin olive oil in a large mixing basin. Refrigerate for around 30 minutes while you prepare the remaining ingredients.
- ➤ Combine the bell pepper, broccoli, carrots, crabmeat, olives, and onion in a mixing bowl. Toss with spaghetti.
- ➤ In a separate bowl, whisk together the mayonnaise, balsamic vinaigrette, Italian seasoning, and black pepper for the dressing, then pour over the pasta salad. To blend, mix everything. Serve at room temperature or chilled, garnished with cherry tomatoes.

Shrimp and Pasta Shell Salad

Preparation Time: 10 minutes
Cooking Time: 15 minutes
Servings: 1

Ingredients:

- One ¼ cups mayonnaise, or more if needed
- Two teaspoons of Dijon mustard
- Two teaspoons ketchup
- ¼ teaspoon Worcestershire sauce
- One teaspoon salt, or to taste
- One pinch of cayenne pepper, or to taste
- One lemon, juiced
- ⅓ cup chopped fresh dill
- Salad:
- 1 (12 ounces) package of small pasta shells
- 1 pound cooked, peeled, and deveined small shrimp - cut in half
- ½ cup finely diced red bell pepper
- ¾ cup diced celery
- salt and ground black pepper to taste
- One pinch of paprika for garnish
- Three sprigs of fresh dill, or as desired

Directions:

- In a mixing bowl, combine 1 1/4 cup mayonnaise, Dijon mustard, ketchup, Worcestershire sauce, salt, and cayenne pepper; add lemon juice and 1/3 cup chopped dill. Whisk until completely blended. Refrigerate.
- Bring a saucepan of salted water to a boil, then add the pasta shells and simmer until cooked, 8 to 10 minutes. Drain and rinse with cold water to slightly chill the pasta; drain again. Transfer to a large mixing bowl.
- Toss shrimp with pasta; toss in red bell pepper, celery, and dressing. Fill shells with a dressing after fully mixing. Refrigerate the bowl for 2 to 3 hours, covered with plastic wrap.
- Before serving, toss the salad with additional salt, black pepper, lemon juice, and cayenne pepper to taste. If the salad feels dry, add a bit of extra mayonnaise. Garnish with paprika and dill sprigs.

Tortellini Pesto Salad

Preparation Time: 10 minutes
Cooking Time: 15 minutes
Servings: 1

Ingredients:

- 1 (9 ounces) package of cheese tortellini
- One small red bell pepper, julienned
- ¾ cup broccoli florets, blanched
- ⅓ cup shredded carrots
- ⅓ cup pitted green olives
- One clove of garlic, chopped
- ½ cup mayonnaise
- ¼ cup prepared basil pesto
- ¼ cup milk
- Two tablespoons of grated Parmesan cheese
- One tablespoon of olive oil
- One tablespoon of distilled white vinegar
- One bunch of fresh spinach leaves

Directions:

- Warm up a big saucepan of gently salted water. Cook for 7 to 8 minutes, or until the tortellini is al dente. Cool after draining.
- Combine the cooked tortellini, red bell pepper, broccoli, carrots, olives, and garlic in a large mixing basin.
- Separately, combine the mayonnaise, pesto, milk, Parmesan cheese, olive oil, and vinegar. Toss the tortellini and veggies in the sauce to coat. Refrigerate for 1 hour, or until cool, covered. Serve on top of spinach leaves.

Kale Fiesta Salad

Preparation Time: 10 minutes
Cooking Time: 15 minutes
Servings: 1

Ingredients:

- Two lemons, juiced, divided
- One bunch of fresh basil leaves, divided
- Two cloves of garlic, crushed and peeled
- Two tablespoons of olive oil, divided
- One tablespoon shredded Parmesan cheese, or to taste
- salt and ground black pepper to taste
- ½ pound skinless, boneless chicken thighs
- One small onion, thinly sliced
- Two tablespoons vinegar
- One tablespoon honey
- 1 (8 ounces) package kale, ribs removed and leaves torn into pieces
- 1 English cucumber, cubed
- One large heirloom tomato, cubed
- One large carrot, cubed
- 1 cup fresh corn kernels
- ½ (15 ounces) can of black beans, rinsed and drained
- ½ (6 ounces) can of black olives

Directions:

- Preheat the oven carefully to 375° F. (190 degrees C).
- In a food processor, combine the juice of half a lemon, half of the basil, garlic, one tablespoon of olive oil, Parmesan cheese, salt, and pepper until smooth. In a nonstick baking pan, place the chicken thighs.
- Thirty minutes in a preheated oven with bare chicken thighs. Remove chicken from the oven and pour the mixed mixture over it.
- Continue baking for another 15 minutes, or until the chicken is no longer pink in the centre and the juices run clear. Allow cooling for 10 minutes. Using two forks, shred the chicken. Place aside.
- In a saucepan over medium-low heat, heat the remaining olive oil. Cook until the onion is cooked and golden brown, about 10 minutes. Combine the remaining lemon juice and basil, vinegar, and honey in a mixing bowl. 5 minutes to completely heat dressing
- Combine the chicken, kale, cucumber, tomato, carrot, corn, black beans, and olives in a mixing bowl.
- Massage and toss salad with warm dressing until fully covered.

Celery Root Salad

Preparation Time: 10 minutes
Cooking Time: 15 minutes
Servings: 1

Ingredients:

- 1 pound celery root
- Three tablespoons of rapeseed oil
- Two tablespoons of lemon juice
- One tablespoon of white wine vinegar
- salt and freshly ground black pepper to taste

Directions:

- Peel and cut the celery root into quarters. Put in a saucepan with moderately salted water. Bring to a boil, lower to low heat, and cook until the potatoes are cooked for about 20 minutes. Drain and keep aside until completely cold. Place in a salad dish and cut into pieces.
- Combine the oil, lemon juice, vinegar, salt, and pepper in a small bowl. The dressing should be poured over celery root. Allow marinating for at least 2 hours to allow flavours to develop.

Mediterranean Salmon Pasta Salad

Preparation Time: 10 minutes
Cooking Time: 15 minutes
Servings: 1

Ingredients:

- ½ (16 ounces) package of mezze (short) penne pasta
- 1 cup sliced and quartered cucumber
- 1 cup halved cherry tomatoes
- Two tablespoons of minced shallot
- 1 (2.6 ounces) pouch of wild-caught pink salmon (such as Chicken of the Sea®)
- Vinaigrette:
- ¼ cup extra-virgin olive oil
- One tablespoon of white wine vinegar
- One tablespoon of freshly squeezed lemon juice
- One teaspoon lemon-pepper seasoning
- ½ teaspoon Dijon mustard
- ½ teaspoon salt
- ¼ teaspoon dried dill weed

Directions:

- ➢ Warm up a big saucepan of gently salted water. Cook, occasionally tossing, until the penne is cooked but still firm to the bite, approximately 10 minutes. Drain, rinse with cold water and serve in a serving dish.
- ➢ Serve spaghetti topped with cucumber, tomatoes, and shallots. Salmon should be broken up and sprinkled on top.
- ➢ In a small mixing bowl, combine the olive oil, vinegar, lemon juice, lemon-pepper spice, mustard, salt, and dill for the vinaigrette. Drizzle over salad and gently mix to incorporate.

Grimm's Grilled Cobb Salad

Preparation Time: 10 minutes
Cooking Time: 15 minutes
Servings: 1

Ingredients:

- Six tablespoons oil, plus more for grilling
- Three tablespoons of red wine vinegar
- One tablespoon of Dijon mustard
- One teaspoon honey
- One clove of garlic, minced
- Salt and pepper
- One large head of green leaf lettuce halved (5 Cup yield)
- Two ripe vine tomatoes halved
- Two firm avocados
- Two ears of corn, whole and cleaned
- One package of Grimm's Bacon and Cheddar Bavarian Smokies
- Four hardboiled eggs, diced
- ½ cup Grimm's Medium Cheddar Cheese, grated
- Grimm's Cheese Tortilla Wraps, grilled. Preheat grill.

Directions:

- ➢ 6 tbsp oil, red wine vinegar, Dijon, honey, and garlic in a small bowl. Set aside and season with salt and pepper.
- ➢ Toss lettuce halves with two tablespoons of oil, salt, and pepper to taste. Toss the tomato halves with two tablespoons of oil, salt, and pepper to taste. Remove the seeds from the avocados and retain them in their shells. Season the avocados on the interior with oil, salt, and pepper. Toss the corn in 2 tablespoons of oil, salt, and pepper.
- ➢ Place the smokies and corn on the grill, charring them outside and cooking them. Next, char the insides of the lettuce, tomatoes, and avocados on high heat, leaving them mostly uncooked. All you want is the burnt flavour.
- ➢ Remove all of the grill's ingredients. Smokies should be cut into half-moons, the tomato should be diced, corn should be removed from the cob, and avocados should be sliced. It's now time to put everything together.

- ➢ Arrange the charred lettuce on a big tray, followed by a row of tomatoes, the hardboiled eggs, the sliced smokies, the Cheddar, the avocados, and corn. Serve with grilled tortillas and the red wine vinaigrette.

Classic Chicken Salad

Preparation Time: 10 minutes
Cooking Time: 15 minutes
Servings: 1

Ingredients:

- cooking spray
- 2 pounds skinless, boneless chicken breast halves
- One teaspoon kosher salt, divided
- ¾ teaspoon ground black pepper, divided
- ¾ teaspoon onion powder
- 1 cup mayonnaise, or more to taste
- ½ cup sour cream
- ¼ cup sweet relish
- Three stalks of green onions (white and light green parts only), minced
- Two tablespoons of chopped fresh parsley
- One tablespoon of Dijon mustard
- One tablespoon of lemon juice
- One teaspoon of dried dill weed
- ½ cup finely chopped celery

Directions:

- ➢ Preheat the oven carefully to 300° F. (150 degrees C). Coat a baking dish lightly with cooking spray.
- ➢ Treat the chicken equally with 1/2 teaspoon salt, 1/2 teaspoon pepper, and onion powder. Cover securely with foil and place in the prepared baking dish.
- ➢ Bake until the juices run clear and the chicken shreds easily, approximately 1 hour 20 minutes; do not overcook. In the middle, an instant-read thermometer should read at least 165 degrees F. (74 degrees C).
- ➢ Remove from the oven, cover, and set aside for 15 minutes or until cool enough to handle. Keep any leftover chicken broth.
- ➢ While the chicken cools, make the dressing. In a large mixing bowl, add 1 cup mayonnaise, sour cream, relish, green onions, parsley, Dijon, lemon juice, dill, and remaining salt and pepper.
- ➢ Place the chicken in the bowl of a food processor in big chunks. To shred the chicken to the appropriate consistency, pulse 3 to 5 times.
- ➢ Place the chicken in a bowl. Pour dressing over celery and toss to coat. If extra moisture is wanted, add more mayonnaise or leftover broth.
- ➢ Before serving, cover and chill for at least 2 hours (or up to 2 days). Before serving, thoroughly combine all ingredients.

Beef Tip Salad Topping

Preparation Time: 10 minutes
Cooking Time: 15 minutes
Servings: 1

Ingredients:

- ½ cup olive oil
- One tablespoon of soy sauce
- One onion, sliced
- One green bell pepper, seeded and thinly sliced
- 1 pound beef stew meat, cut into 1/2 inch pieces

Directions:

- ➢ In a large pan over medium heat, heat the olive oil. Combine the soy sauce, onion, and green bell pepper in a mixing bowl—Cook for 3 to 5 minutes, or until the vegetables are soft. Stir in the beef stew meat. Cook, stirring regularly, for 15 minutes or until uniformly browned.

Summer Grilled Shrimp Salad

Preparation Time: 10 minutes
Cooking Time: 15 minutes
Servings: 1

Ingredients:

- One tablespoon of olive oil
- Two ¼ teaspoons of smokehouse maple seasoning (such as McCormick® Grill Mates®)
- 1 ½ teaspoon lemon juice
- 12 ounces peeled and deveined shrimp
- Cilantro Vinaigrette:
- ¼ cup extra-virgin olive oil
- Two tablespoons honey
- Two tablespoons of fresh lime juice
- Two tablespoons of chopped cilantro
- One tablespoon of balsamic vinegar
- salt and ground black pepper to taste
- Salad:
- 4 cups mixed salad greens, or more to taste
- ½ cup thinly sliced English cucumber
- ⅓ cup freshly cooked corn
- ½ cup diced tomato
- ¼ cup sliced red onion
- One avocado, diced

Directions:

- ➤ Combine the olive oil, maple seasoning, and lemon juice in a glass bowl. Toss in the shrimp to coat. Refrigerate until ready to cook on the grill.
- ➤ Combine the olive oil, honey, lime juice, cilantro, balsamic vinegar, salt, and pepper in a small mixing bowl. Set aside the vinaigrette.
- ➤ Preheat a medium-high grill, either indoors or outside. Thread the shrimp onto skewers and serve. Grill the shrimp until they are pink and opaque, about 2 minutes on each side. Set aside after removing off skewers.
- ➤ Fill a large salad dish halfway with mixed greens. On top of the greens, arrange cucumber, corn, tomato, red onion, and avocado in slices. Arrange the grilled shrimp in the salad's middle. Drizzle the vinaigrette over the salad and toss to coat. Serve right away.

Southwest Layered Salad

Preparation Time: 10 minutes
Cooking Time: 15 minutes
Servings: 1

Ingredients:

- 1 (1 ounce) package of dry ranch dressing mix (such as Hidden Valley Ranch®)
- 1 cup buttermilk
- 1 cup fat-free plain yoghurt
- ½ (1.25 ounce) package of taco seasoning mix, or more to taste
- Salad:
- 8 cups torn romaine lettuce
- Two roasted red peppers, diced
- 1 (14 ounces) can of black beans, rinsed and drained
- 1 (14 ounces) can of white corn, drained
- ¼ cup finely chopped sweet onion
- 1 (4 ounces) can dice green chile peppers
- 1 cup diced Roma tomatoes
- ½ cup shredded sharp Cheddar cheese
- One large avocado - peeled, pitted, and sliced
- ¼ cup chopped fresh cilantro (optional)

Directions:

- ➤ Combine the dressing mix, buttermilk, yoghurt, and taco seasoning mix in a bowl.
- ➤ Toss the lettuce into a large serving basin.
- ➤ Combine roasted peppers, black beans, corn, onion, and green chiles in a mixing bowl. Spread the mixture on top of

the lettuce. Sprinkle with Cheddar cheese and top with tomatoes. Arrange avocado slices in a circle, overlapping them. Garnish with cilantro if desired. The dressing should be served on the side.

Buffalo Chicken Mason Jar Salads

Preparation Time: 10 minutes
Cooking Time: 15 minutes
Servings: 1

Ingredients:

- 10 ounces cucumber ranch salad dressing
- Two tablespoons Buffalo-style hot pepper sauce (such as Frank's® RedHot)
- Four stalks of celery, cut into 1/8-inch slices
- Four medium carrots, cut into 1/8-inch slices
- 15 ounces cooked chicken, cut into bite-sized pieces
- 10 cups salad greens
- One ¼ cup crumbled blue cheese
- ¾ cup croutons (Optional)

Directions:

- ➤ In a small bowl, combine ranch dressing and spicy sauce. Form the first layer by dividing the dressing evenly among five wide-mouthed, quart-sized glass canning jars. Form the next two layers with equal amounts of celery and carrots.
- ➤ Fill each jar with 3 ounces of chicken. Top the chicken with 2 cups of salad greens in each jar—top salad greens with 1/4 cup blue cheese. Refrigerate the jars until ready to use.
- ➤ Divide the croutons evenly into five small covered containers. Toss the jar contents and croutons into a bowl when ready to dine.

Amy's Barbecue Chicken Salad

Preparation Time: 10 minutes
Cooking Time: 15 minutes
Servings: 1

Ingredients:

- Two skinless, boneless chicken breast halves
- One head of red leaf lettuce, rinsed and torn
- One head of green leaf lettuce, rinsed and torn
- One fresh tomato, chopped
- One bunch of cilantro, chopped
- 1 (15.25 ounce) can of whole kernel corn, drained
- 1 (15 ounces) can of black beans, drained
- 1 (2.8 ounces) can French fried onions
- ½ cup Ranch dressing
- ½ cup barbeque sauce

Directions:

- ➤ Preheat the grill to high.
- ➤ Oil the grill grate lightly. Grill the chicken for 6 minutes per side or until the juices run clear. Remove from the flame, allow it cool, and then slice.
- ➤ Combine the red leaf lettuce, green leaf lettuce, tomato, cilantro, corn, and black beans in a large mixing basin. Serve with grilled chicken chunks and French fried onions on top.
- ➤ Combine the Ranch dressing and barbecue sauce in a small bowl. Serve as a dipping sauce on the side, or mix with the salad to coat.

Simple Red Leaf Salad

Preparation Time: 10 minutes
Cooking Time: 15 minutes
Servings: 1

Ingredients:

- One head of red leaf lettuce
- One red bell pepper, chopped
- One stalk of green onion, thinly sliced
- Dressing:

- Three tablespoons extra-virgin olive oil
- One tablespoon of red wine vinegar
- One tablespoon of balsamic vinegar
- One tablespoon of lemon juice
- ½ teaspoon salt, or to taste
- ¼ teaspoon Dijon mustard, or more to taste
- freshly ground black pepper to taste

Directions:
- ➤ Wash and separate the leaves of red leaf lettuce with a salad spinner. Tear the leaves into bite-sized pieces and combine with the bell pepper and scallions in a salad dish.
- ➤ Combine olive oil, red wine vinegar, balsamic vinegar, lemon juice, salt, mustard, and pepper in a resealable container. Close and shake until well blended.
- ➤ Drizzle the salad with as much dressing as desired and toss to incorporate. Keep any remaining dressing in the fridge.

Spicy English Seven-Layer Salad

Preparation Time: 10 minutes
Cooking Time: 15 minutes
Servings: 1

Ingredients:
- 2 cups small seashell pasta
- Four carrots, peeled and julienned
- ½ head leaf lettuce - rinsed, dried, and chopped
- One medium cucumber, peeled, seeded, and diced
- ¾ cup frozen green peas
- ½ cup frozen whole-kernel corn
- 2 cups mayonnaise
- Two tablespoons of brown sugar
- One tablespoon of curry powder
- ½ teaspoon garlic salt
- 1 cup shredded Cheddar cheese

Directions:
- ➤ Warm-up a saucepan of gently salted water. Cook until the pasta is cooked, about 7 minutes. To cool, drain and rinse with cold water.
- ➤ Make a uniform layer of carrots in the bottom of a big glass bowl, preferably one that is nearly the same diameter from top to bottom. Arrange the lettuce on top of the carrots. Spread the cucumber, peas, and corn in a layer over the lettuce. Once the spaghetti has cooled and been drained, distribute it over the top.

- ➤ Combine the mayonnaise, brown sugar, curry powder, and garlic salt in a separate small bowl. Carefully spread this over the spaghetti—shredded Cheddar cheese on top. Refrigerate for at least 1 hour before serving, covered.

Rice Salad

Preparation Time: 10 minutes
Cooking Time: 15 minutes
Servings: 1

Ingredients:
- 2 cups water
- 1 cup white rice
- Six eggs
- 1 (10 ounces) package of frozen peas, thawed
- 1 cup chopped celery
- ¼ cup chopped onion
- 1 (4 ounces) jar diced pimento
- 1 cup mayonnaise
- One teaspoon of prepared mustard
- One tablespoon of lemon juice
- ¼ cup sweet pickle relish
- 1 (9 ounces) can of solid white tuna packed in water, drained
- ¼ teaspoon dried dill weed
- One teaspoon salt
- ⅛ teaspoon pepper

Directions:
- ➤ Bring water to a boil in a saucepan. Stir in the rice. Reduce the heat to low, cover, and cook for 20 minutes. Remove from the heat and leave to cool.
- ➤ Cover the eggs in a saucepan with cold water. Bring to a boil and then remove from heat. Allow eggs to stand in boiling water for 10 to 12 minutes, covered. Remove from the boiling water, and allow to cool before peeling and chopping.
- ➤ Cold water should be used to rinse frozen peas. Place in a large mixing basin after straining. Toss in the eggs, rice, celery, onions, and pimiento. In a separate mixing bowl, combine the mayonnaise, mustard, lemon juice, relish, tuna, dill, salt, and pepper until thoroughly combined. Toss with the veggie mixture to incorporate. Refrigerate for at least 4 hours, covered. Before serving, toss once more. Chill before serving.

CHAPTER 19: SNACKS

Cheese Wizards

Preparation Time: 10 minutes
Cooking Time: 15 minutes
Servings: 1

Ingredients:

- 1 pound lean ground beef
- 1 (16 ounces) jar of processed cheese sauce
- salt and pepper to taste
- 16 ounces cocktail rye bread

Directions:

➢ Preheat the oven carefully to broil.
➢ In a big, deep-pan, brown the ground meat. Cook until uniformly browned over medium-high heat. Drain and break the bread.
➢ Combine the meat, processed cheese sauce, salt, and pepper in a medium mixing bowl. Spread the mixture on the cocktail rye pieces.
➢ Broil the slices for 5 minutes, or until the cheese sauce has melted, on a large baking sheet.

Midnight Snack Avocado Sandwich

Preparation Time: 10 minutes
Cooking Time: 15 minutes
Servings: 1

Ingredients:

- Two slices of bacon, cut into 1-inch pieces
- Two green onions, chopped
- One tablespoon mayonnaise
- Two slices of whole-wheat bread, toasted
- ½ avocado, mashed
- Three slices tomato
- ⅓ cup alfalfa sprouts
- salt and ground black pepper to taste

Directions:

➢ Cook the bacon in a large pan over medium-high heat, rotating periodically, for 2 to 3 minutes, or until nearly browned. Cook and stir until the green onion is tender and the bacon is crisp, 3 to 5 minutes more.
➢ On one side of each slice of bread, spread mayonnaise. On one slice of bread, spread mashed avocado on one side. Top with tomato slices, sprouts, and bacon combination; season with salt and black pepper to taste. Place the last slice of bread on top.

White Chocolate Snack Mix

Preparation Time: 10 minutes
Cooking Time: 15 minutes
Servings: 1

Ingredients:

- 1 (10 ounces) package mini twist pretzels
- 5 cups toasted oat cereal
- 5 cups crispy corn cereal squares
- 2 cups salted peanuts
- 1 (14 ounces) package of candy-coated milk chocolate pieces
- 2 (11 ounces) packages of white chocolate chips
- Three tablespoons of vegetable oil

Directions:

➢ Line three baking sheets with parchment or greased paper. Place aside.
➢ In a large mixing dish, combine micro pretzels, toasted oat cereal, crispy corn cereal squares, salted peanuts, and candy-coated chocolate pieces. Place aside.

➢ Microwave chips and oil in a microwave-safe bowl for 2 minutes, stirring once. Microwave for 10 seconds on high, then whisk until smooth. Pour over the cereal mixture and thoroughly combine.
➢ Distribute evenly on prepared baking sheets. Allow cooling before separating. Keep it in an airtight container.

Crunchy Chocolate Chip Peanut Butter Snack Bites

Preparation Time: 10 minutes
Cooking Time: 15 minutes
Servings: 1

Ingredients:

- 1 cup large flake rolled oats
- ½ cup KRAFT Crunchy Peanut Butter
- ¼ cup honey
- ½ cup salted peanuts, chopped
- ½ cup BAKER'S Semi-Sweet Chocolate Chips

Directions:

➢ In a medium mixing bowl, combine all ingredients until well combined. Refrigerate for 20–30 minutes.
➢ Roll into 20 (1-inch) balls, about two tablespoons each.

Sweet and Crunchy Popcorn Snack Mix

Preparation Time: 10 minutes
Cooking Time: 15 minutes
Servings: 1

Ingredients:

- waxed paper
- 2 cups crispy corn and rice cereal (such as Crispix®)
- 2 cups honey graham cereal (such as Golden Grahams®)
- 2 cups peanut butter corn puff cereal (such as Reese's Puffs®)
- 2 cups popped popcorn, or more to taste (Optional)
- 8 ounces candy-coated milk chocolate pieces (such as M&M's®)
- 1 cup salted peanuts
- ½ cup butter
- Two tablespoons of all-purpose flour
- 1 cup brown sugar
- ½ cup corn syrup
- ½ cup peanut butter

Directions:

➢ The waxed paper should be used to line a big baking sheet.
➢ In a large mixing bowl, combine crunchy corn and rice cereal, honey graham cereal, peanut butter corn puff cereal, popcorn, chocolate bits, and peanuts.
➢ In a large saucepan over medium heat, melt the butter; stir in the flour until smooth, 2 to 3 minutes. Bring brown sugar and corn syrup to a boil, occasionally stirring, for about 1 minute, or until sugar is dissolved. Stir peanut butter into sugar mixture for 3 minutes, or until smooth; pour over cereal mixture and gently toss until coated.
➢ Allow cereal mixture to cool for 30 minutes on a prepared baking sheet. When the mixture has cooled, split it into bits and store it in an airtight container.

Chinese Popcorn Snack Mix

Preparation Time: 10 minutes
Cooking Time: 15 minutes
Servings: 1

Ingredients:

- 10 cups plain popped popcorn, unsalted
- 1 ½ cups chow mein noodles
- 1 cup honey roasted peanuts
- Three tablespoons of unsalted butter, melted
- Two tablespoons of low-sodium soy sauce
- One tablespoon of freshly squeezed lime juice
- 1 ½ teaspoon sesame oil
- One teaspoon of Sriracha sauce, or to taste
- One teaspoon of ground ginger

Directions:
- Preheat the oven carefully to 250° F. (120 degrees C). Aluminium foil or parchment paper should line a large baking sheet.
- Combine the popcorn, chow mein noodles, and peanuts in a large mixing bowl.
- Combine the butter, soy sauce, lime juice, sesame oil, Sriracha, and ginger in a small mixing bowl. Drizzle the butter mixture over the popcorn and toss to coat evenly. Distribute equally on the baking sheet that has been prepared.
- Bake for 30 minutes, stirring halfway through, in a preheated oven. Remove the baking sheet from the oven. Allow cooling before transferring to an airtight container.

Snack Factory® Pretzel Crisps® with Creamy Spinach Dip

Preparation Time: 10 minutes
Cooking Time: 15 minutes
Servings: 1

Ingredients:
- 1 ½ tablespoon olive oil
- One onion, minced
- Two cloves of garlic, minced
- 1 (10 ounces) package frozen chopped spinach, thawed and drained
- ½ cup milk
- 1 (8 ounces) package of cream cheese, softened
- ¼ cup mayonnaise
- 1 cup Parmesan cheese
- Salt and pepper to taste
- 1 (7.2 ounces) package Snack Factory® Original Pretzel Crisps®

Directions:
- Heat the olive oil and sauté the onions and garlic until golden brown in a large saucepan. Season with salt and pepper before adding the spinach.
- Stir in the milk, cream cheese, mayonnaise, and Parmesan cheese until equally combined. Turn the heat down low. Allow the ingredients to cook together while stirring periodically.
- With Snack Factory®, Pretzel Crisps®, serve warm.

Quick Lotus Seed and Nut Snack

Preparation Time: 10 minutes
Cooking Time: 15 minutes
Servings: 1

Ingredients:
- One tablespoon of ghee (clarified butter)
- ⅓ cup cashews
- ½ cup salted peanuts
- 2 cups lotus seeds
- salt and freshly ground black pepper

Directions:
- Heat the ghee in a pan over medium heat and shallow-fry the cashew nuts until aromatic and gently toasted, 2 to 3 minutes. Remove from the skillet and pat dry with paper towels. Fry the peanuts in the same pan for 2 to 3 minutes, or until gently toasted. Fry the lotus seeds over low heat for approximately 3 minutes, or until they are crisp and have absorbed all of the ghee.
- Season cashews, peanuts, and lotus seeds in a dish with salt and pepper. To keep them from getting soggy, store them in an airtight jar.

Heart-y Antioxidant Almond Snack Mix

Preparation Time: 10 minutes
Cooking Time: 15 minutes
Servings: 1

Ingredients:
- 3 cups multi-grain cereal squares, such as Chex® brand
- 3 cups fibre cereal twigs, such as Fiber One® brand
- 1 cup sweetened dried cranberries
- ¾ cup dark chocolate morsels
- ¾ cup almond butter
- ½ cup enriched margarine spread, such as Smart Balance® brand (may use butter)
- ¾ cup almond flour
- ¼ cup sliced almonds
- ¾ cup confectioners' sugar

Directions:
- Line a large baking sheet with waxed paper. In a large resealable plastic bag, combine cereal and dried cranberries. Combine chocolate chips, almond butter, and enhanced margarine spread in a microwave-safe bowl (or butter). Microwave on High for 1 minute, uncovered. Stir. Microwave for 30 seconds more; remove and stir until smooth.
- Fill a plastic bag halfway with the chocolate mixture, seal it, and shake to cover evenly. Combine almond flour, sliced almonds, and confectioners' sugar in a mixing bowl. Shake to coat and reseal. Allow the mixture to cool fully on waxed paper. Refrigerate in an airtight container; the mixture can be kept for a week.

Gabe's Buffalo Ranch Snack Mix

Preparation Time: 10 minutes
Cooking Time: 15 minutes
Servings: 1

Ingredients:
- aluminium foil
- nonstick cooking spray
- 4 cups crispy rice cereal squares (such as Rice Chex®)
- 3 cups crispy corn cereal squares (such as Corn Chex®)
- 3 cups hot and spicy cheese-flavoured crackers (such as Cheez-Its®)
- 2 cups Buffalo-flavored pretzel pieces
- Six tablespoons of butter, melted
- Three tablespoons of hot sauce (such as Frank's® RedHot®)
- 1 (1 ounce) package of dry ranch dressing mix
- ¾ teaspoon celery seed

Directions:
- Preheat the oven carefully to 250° F. (120 degrees C). Spray a large baking sheet with cooking spray and line with aluminium foil.
- In a large mixing bowl, combine rice and corn cereal squares, cheese-flavoured crackers, and pretzel bites.
- In a small mixing bowl, blend the melted butter, hot sauce, ranch dressing, and celery seed until smooth and thoroughly incorporated. Pour over cereal mixture and toss to coat evenly. Spread in an equal layer on the prepared baking sheet.
- 25 to 30 minutes in a preheated oven, stirring every 10 minutes, until crisp. Allow cooling fully after removing from the oven.

Pretzel Broomstick

Preparation Time: 10 minutes
Cooking Time: 15 minutes
Servings: 1

Ingredients:
- Four-string cheese sticks, or more as needed
- 12 pretzel sticks
- One leaf of fresh spinach, cut into strips, or more as needed

Directions:
➢ Each string cheese stick should be cut into thirds. Make thin threads out of the ends of each third to resemble a broom.
➢ To make the broom handle, insert a pretzel stick into each piece of string cheese. Then, wrap the cheese in a spinach strip.

Kerri's Concoction Sweet Snack Mix

Preparation Time: 10 minutes
Cooking Time: 15 minutes
Servings: 1

Ingredients:
- ½ cup butter
- Three tablespoons of brown sugar
- 1 ½ teaspoon ground cinnamon
- One teaspoon of ground ginger
- ½ teaspoon ground nutmeg
- 4 cups toasted oat cereal (such as Cheerios®)
- 4 cups shredded wheat cereal biscuits
- 4 cups crispy rice cereal squares (such as Rice Chex®)
- 2 cups mini pretzels
- 2 cups mixed nuts
- 1 (6 ounces) package of dried cranberries
- 1 (12 ounces) package of white chocolate morsels

Directions:
➢ Preheat the oven carefully to 250°F (120 degrees C).
➢ In a large roasting pan over medium heat, melt the butter. Melt the butter and stir in the brown sugar, cinnamon, ginger, and nutmeg. Stir in the toasted oat cereal, shredded wheat biscuits, rice cereal squares, pretzels, and nuts to cover.
➢ One hour in a preheated oven, stirring every 15 minutes. Set aside to cool before transferring to a large mixing basin.
➢ Fold in the white chocolate morsels and dried cranberries; spread onto a big sheet of waxed paper to chill fully.

Cyd's Christmas Snack

Preparation Time: 10 minutes
Cooking Time: 15 minutes
Servings: 1

Ingredients:
- 1 (12 ounces) package of crispy corn and rice cereal (such as Crispix®)
- ½ cup butter
- Two tablespoons of Worcestershire sauce
- Two teaspoons of hot pepper sauce (such as Tabasco®)
- Two teaspoons of Cajun seasoning
- Two teaspoons of onion powder
- One teaspoon of seasoned salt
- One teaspoon of garlic powder

Directions:
➢ Preheat the oven carefully to 250°F (120 degrees C).
➢ Fill a big roasting pan halfway with cereal.
➢ In a microwave-safe bowl, melt the butter for about 90 seconds. Combine Worcestershire sauce, spicy pepper sauce, Cajun spice, onion powder, seasoned salt, and garlic powder in a mixing bowl. Pour the mixture over the cereal and coat evenly.
➢ Toss every 15 minutes in a hot oven until crispy, about 1 hour. Allow cooling.

Easy Snack Wraps

Preparation Time: 10 minutes
Cooking Time: 15 minutes
Servings: 1

Ingredients:
- 12 (10 inches) flour tortillas
- 1 (8 ounces) package of cream cheese
- One head lettuce
- 1 (6 ounces) package of sliced deli-style turkey
- 2 cups shredded carrots
- 2 cups minced tomato

Directions:
➢ Cover the tortillas equally with cream cheese. Place lettuce leaves on top of the cream cheese. Arrange the turkey slices on top of the lettuce in uniform layers. Sprinkle the carrots and tomato slices on top of the turkey pieces. Make wraps out of the tortillas. Cut the wraps into bite-sized pieces by cutting them diagonally. Use toothpicks to secure.

Caramel Snack Mix

Preparation Time: 10 minutes
Cooking Time: 15 minutes
Servings: 1

Ingredients:
- ½ cup butter
- ¾ cup white corn syrup
- 1 cup packed brown sugar
- 1 cup chopped pecans
- 1 cup almonds
- 1 (12 ounces) package of crispy corn and rice cereal

Directions:
➢ Preheat the oven carefully to 275°F (135 degrees C). I am using nonstick cooking spray and coating a large roasting pan.
➢ Combine butter, white corn syrup, and brown sugar in a medium microwave-safe bowl—Microwave the mixture for 2 minutes or until the butter melts.
➢ Fill the roasting pan halfway with cereal, pecans, and almonds. Pour the melted butter mixture over the cereal and almonds and gently stir until evenly covered.
➢ 1 hour in the oven, stirring every 15 minutes
➢ Continue to stir the snack mix as it cools so that it does not solidify into one huge lump.

Maple Apple Pie Protein Squares

Preparation Time: 10 minutes
Cooking Time: 15 minutes
Servings: 1

Ingredients:
- 1 cup unsweetened applesauce
- ¾ cup maple syrup
- ½ cup crunchy almond butter
- 4 cups oat flour
- Two tablespoons of ground cinnamon
- Two tablespoons of unsweetened cocoa powder
- Two scoops of vanilla-flavoured whey protein powder

Directions:
➢ Using parchment paper, line a 9x13-inch baking dish.
➢ In a large mixing dish, combine applesauce, maple syrup, and almond butter. Mix the oat flour, cinnamon, chocolate, and protein powder until thoroughly blended. Spread the mixture into the prepared dish.
➢ Refrigerate for 1 hour or until firm. Wrap with parchment paper and cut into 30 squares.

Blueberry Zucchini Muffins

Preparation Time: 10 minutes
Cooking Time: 15 minutes
Servings: 1

Ingredients:

- 1 ½ cups all-purpose flour
- ½ cup white sugar
- ¼ cup brown sugar
- One teaspoon of baking soda
- One teaspoon of ground cinnamon
- ½ teaspoon salt
- ½ cup olive oil
- ¼ cup milk
- One egg
- 1 ½ teaspoons vanilla extract
- 1 cup shredded zucchini
- ½ cup fresh blueberries
- ½ cup chopped pecans

Directions:

- ➢ Preheat the oven carefully to 350°F (175 degrees C). Grease or line 12 muffin cups with paper liners.
- ➢ Combine the flour, white sugar, brown sugar, baking soda, cinnamon, and salt in a mixing dish. In a separate bowl, whisk the olive oil, milk, egg, and vanilla extract until smooth; fold into the flour mixture until moistened. Mix in the zucchini, blueberries, and pecans. 2/3 fill prepared muffin cups with batter.
- ➢ Bake for 20 to 25 minutes, or until a toothpick inserted into the middle of a muffin comes out clean.

Oatmeal Chocolate Chip Snack Bars

Preparation Time: 10 minutes
Cooking Time: 15 minutes
Servings: 1

Ingredients:

- ½ cup unsweetened applesauce
- ¼ cup packed brown sugar
- Two tablespoons of white sugar
- One egg white
- One tablespoon of canola oil
- One tablespoon milk
- One teaspoon of vanilla extract
- ¾ cup whole wheat flour
- ½ teaspoon baking soda
- ½ teaspoon ground cinnamon
- ⅛ teaspoon salt
- 1 ½ cup rolled oats
- ½ cup chocolate chips

Directions:

- ➢ Preheat the oven carefully to 350° F. (175 degrees C).
- ➢ Combine the applesauce, brown sugar, white sugar, egg white, oil, milk, and vanilla extract in a mixing bowl.

- ➢ In a separate basin, combine the flour, baking soda, cinnamon, and salt; add to the applesauce mixture. Combine the oats and chocolate chips in a mixing bowl. Spread the dough in an oiled 9x13-inch baking pan.
- ➢ 20 to 25 minutes in a preheated oven until golden brown. Allow cooling fully before slicing into 16 bars.

Beer Cheese Dip from Snack Factory®

Preparation Time: 10 minutes
Cooking Time: 15 minutes
Servings: 1

Ingredients:

- 8 ounces shredded Cheddar cheese
- 6 ounces cream cheese, softened
- Two cloves of garlic, diced
- ½ cup beer
- Two teaspoons cornstarch
- Paprika
- 1 (7.2 ounces) package Original Snack Factory® Pretzel Crisps®

Directions:

- ➢ Preheat the oven carefully to 375°F (190 degrees C). Spray a glass baking dish lightly with nonstick cooking spray.
- ➢ Combine the shredded cheese, softened cream cheese, garlic cloves, and beer in a food processor. Blend until smooth and blended. Process a bit further to incorporate the cornstarch and paprika. Spread the mixture into the prepared baking dish.
- ➢ Bake until bubbly, about 35 minutes, in a preheated oven. Serve with Pretzel Crisps® from Snack Factory®.

Sugar Coated Pecans

Preparation Time: 10 minutes
Cooking Time: 15 minutes
Servings: 1

Ingredients:

- One egg white
- One tablespoon water
- 1 pound of pecan halves
- 1 cup white sugar
- ¾ teaspoon salt
- ½ teaspoon ground cinnamon

Directions:

- ➢ Preheat the oven carefully to 250°F (120 degrees C). One baking sheet should be greased.
- ➢ Whip the egg white and water together in a mixing basin until foamy. Separately, combine the sugar, salt, and cinnamon.
- ➢ Add pecans to egg whites and swirl to coat evenly. Toss the nuts in the sugar mixture until evenly coated. Arrange the nuts on the prepared baking sheet.
- ➢ One hour at 250 degrees F (120 degrees C). Every 15 minutes, stir.

CHAPTER 20: DESSERTS

Cappuccino Truffle Dessert

Preparation Time: 10 minutes
Cooking Time: 15 minutes
Servings: 1

Ingredients:

- Four teaspoons of instant coffee granules
- One tablespoon of hot water
- 1 ½ cups milk
- 1 (3.9 ounces) package of instant chocolate pudding mix
- ½ teaspoon ground cinnamon
- 1 (8 ounces) container whipped cream topping (such as Cool Whip®)
- 1 (9 inches) angel food cake, cubed

Directions:

- ➢ In a large mixing basin, dissolve instant coffee in boiling water. Pour in the milk, pudding mix, and cinnamon. Allow standing for 5 minutes.
- ➢ Gently fold in the whipped topping. Before serving, place a few cake pieces in a dessert bowl and top with chocolate truffle cream.

Quick and Easy Lemon Pineapple Dessert

Preparation Time: 10 minutes
Cooking Time: 15 minutes
Servings: 1

Ingredients:

- 1 (6 ounces) container of nonfat vanilla yoghurt
- 1 (6 ounces) container of nonfat lemon yoghurt
- 1 (8 ounces) can crush pineapple, drained
- 1 (1 ounce) package of fat-free, sugar-free lemon pudding mix (such as Jell-O®)
- 1 cup low-fat frozen whipped topping (such as Cool Whip® Lite), thawed
- Four teaspoons of toasted coconut (Optional)
- Four fresh blueberries (Optional)

Directions:

- ➢ Add vanilla yoghurt, lemon yoghurt, pineapple, and pudding mix; stir until thoroughly blended. Whip in the whipped topping.
- ➢ Fill four dessert bowls with the mixture and refrigerate for 30 minutes.
- ➢ If preferred, garnish each dish with a blueberry, toasted coconut, or an additional dollop of whipped topping.

Toffee Dessert

Preparation Time: 10 minutes
Cooking Time: 15 minutes
Servings: 1

Ingredients:

- 1 (1.4 ounces) bar chocolate-covered toffee
- 1 (1.6 ounces) bar chocolate-covered crispy peanut butter flavoured candy
- 1 cup crushed saltine crackers
- 2 cups crushed graham crackers
- ½ cup butter, melted
- 1 (5.1 ounces) package of instant vanilla pudding mix
- 1 (5.9 ounces) package of instant chocolate pudding mix
- 2 cups milk
- 1 (12 ounces) container of frozen whipped topping, thawed
- 1 (8 ounces) container of frozen whipped topping, thawed

Directions:

- ➢ Freeze the chocolate-covered toffee bar and chocolate-covered crispy peanut butter-flavoured candy bar for 8 hours or overnight.
- ➢ Combine the saltine crackers, graham crackers, and melted butter in a medium mixing basin. To produce a crust, press the mixture into the bottom of a 9x13 inch pan. Refrigerate the crust while you prepare the filling.
- ➢ Combine the instant vanilla pudding mix, instant chocolate pudding mix, and milk in a large mixing basin. Twelve ounces froze whipped topping, folded in. Spread the prepared crust with the filling. Cover the leftover frozen whipped topping with the filling.
- ➢ Crush the frozen chocolate-covered toffee and chocolate-covered crunchy peanut butter candy bars. Crush the candy bars and sprinkle them over the dessert. Refrigerate until ready to serve, covered.

Frosty Strawberry Dessert

Preparation Time: 10 minutes
Cooking Time: 15 minutes
Servings: 1

Ingredients:

- 1 cup all-purpose flour
- ¼ cup brown sugar
- ½ cup chopped walnuts
- ½ cup melted butter or margarine
- Two egg whites
- 1 cup white sugar
- 2 cups sliced strawberries
- Two tablespoons of lemon juice
- 1 cup whipped cream

Directions:

- ➢ Preheat the oven carefully to 350°F (175 degrees C).
- ➢ Combine the flour, brown sugar, walnuts, and melted butter in a mixing dish. Spread out on a baking sheet and bake for 20 minutes, or until crispy, then remove from the oven and cool completely.
- ➢ Beat the egg whites to soft peaks, then beat to stiff peaks while gradually adding the sugar. Toss the strawberries with the lemon juice and fold them into the egg whites until they are slightly pink. Finally, fold in the whipped cream until well combined.
- ➢ Crumble the walnut mixture and evenly distribute it to the bottom of a 9x13 inch dish. Spread the strawberry mixture over the crumbs, then top with the remaining crumbs. Place in the freezer for two hours or until firm. Remove from the freezer a few minutes before serving to make slicing easier.

Plum Dessert

Preparation Time: 10 minutes
Cooking Time: 15 minutes
Servings: 1

Ingredients:

- butter-flavoured cooking spray
- 2 pounds plums
- One teaspoon vanilla sugar, or as needed
- ⅔ cup vanilla sugar
- ½ cup unbleached all-purpose flour
- One tablespoon of butter-flavoured granules
- ½ teaspoon baking powder
- ½ teaspoon ground cinnamon
- ½ teaspoon salt
- ¾ cup fresh orange juice
- ¼ cup liquid egg substitute

- Two tablespoons of canola oil

Directions:
- ➢ Preheat the oven carefully to 350° F. (175 degrees C). Coat a 7x11-inch baking dish liberally with cooking spray.
- ➢ Slice plums without peeling and discard pits. Toss plums in a bowl with one teaspoon of vanilla sugar, depending on how sweet they are. Place aside.
- ➢ In a large mixing basin, combine 2/3 cup vanilla sugar, flour, butter granules, baking powder, cinnamon, and salt. Stir until well combined.
- ➢ In a 2-cup liquid measure, whisk orange juice and liquid egg until fully combined. Mix with the oil. Pour into the dry ingredients and whisk until well combined but not overworked. Cover with sugared plums in the prepared baking dish.
- ➢ 55 to 60 minutes in a preheated oven until the cake is brown and the plums are soft and delicious.
- ➢ Allow cooling for 30 minutes after removing from the oven. Cut into 12 pieces to serve.

Most Delish Quick Dessert In the Universe

Preparation Time: 10 minutes
Cooking Time: 15 minutes
Servings: 1

Ingredients:
- One sweet potato, cooked and mashed
- ¼ teaspoon ground cinnamon, or to taste
- ¼ cup chopped pecans (optional)
- One tablespoon of honey or more to taste

Directions:
- ➢ In a microwave-safe dish, place the mashed sweet potato. If using, stir in the cinnamon and pecans. Drizzle with honey to finish.
- ➢ Heat in the microwave until warm. Serve right away.

Blueberry Cream Dessert

Preparation Time: 10 minutes
Cooking Time: 15 minutes
Servings: 1

Ingredients:
- One ¼ cup of graham cracker crumbs
- Six tablespoons of butter, melted
- ¼ cup white sugar
- Blueberry Cream:
- ¾ cup cold water
- ½ cup white sugar
- 1 (.25 ounce) package of unflavored gelatin
- 1 cup sour cream
- 1 (8 ounces) container of blueberry-flavoured yoghurt
- ½ teaspoon vanilla extract
- ½ cup heavy whipping cream
- 1 cup blueberries

Directions:
- ➢ Combine graham cracker crumbs, melted butter, and 1/4 cup white sugar in a mixing dish. Set aside 1/4 cup of the crust mixture. Fill a 10x6x2-inch baking pan halfway with the remaining crust mixture.
- ➢ In a saucepan over medium-low heat, combine water, 1/2 cup white sugar, and gelatin; boil and stir for 5 minutes until gelatin and sugar dissolve.
- ➢ In a mixing dish, combine the sour cream and yoghurt. Stir gelatin mixture into the sour cream mixture gradually; add vanilla extract. Refrigerate for 30 minutes or until almost set.
- ➢ Whip heavy cream into a glass or metal mixing bowl until soft peaks form. Fold whipped cream into sour cream mixture; whisk in blueberries. Spread blueberry cream evenly over crust; top with leftover 1/4 graham cracker mixture. Refrigerate for 8 hours to overnight.

Pumpkin Pie Dessert Hummus

Preparation Time: 10 minutes
Cooking Time: 15 minutes
Servings: 1

Ingredients:
- 1 (15 ounces) can of chickpeas, drained
- ½ cup canned pumpkin
- Three pitted Medjool dates
- Three tablespoons of maple syrup
- Two tablespoons of unsweetened peanut butter
- One tablespoon diced fresh ginger
- One tablespoon molasses
- One tablespoon of vanilla extract
- 1 ½ teaspoon ground cinnamon
- ¼ teaspoon ground cloves
- ¼ teaspoon ground nutmeg

Directions:
- ➢ In a food processor, combine chickpeas, pumpkin, dates, maple syrup, peanut butter, ginger, molasses, vanilla essence, cinnamon, cloves, and nutmeg. For 2 to 3 minutes, we scraped down sides as needed, the process to a smooth paste. Then, 1 to 2 hours before serving, place in the refrigerator.

Shot Glass Cream Cheese Dessert

Preparation Time: 10 minutes
Cooking Time: 15 minutes
Servings: 1

Ingredients:
- ½ cup miniature chocolate chips
- 2 (8 ounces) packages of cream cheese
- ¾ cup white sugar
- 1 ½ cups chocolate chips
- 12 milk chocolate candy kisses (such as Hershey's Kisses®) (Optional)

Directions:
- ➢ Fill 12 shot glasses halfway with small chocolate chips.
- ➢ In a mixing bowl, use an electric hand mixer on medium speed to combine the cream cheese and sugar.
- ➢ Alternate layers of cream cheese and chocolate chips in the shot glasses. Garnish with milk chocolate candy kisses if desired.

Strawberry Salad Dessert

Preparation Time: 10 minutes

Cooking Time: 15 minutes
Servings: 1

Ingredients:
- 1 (18.25 ounce) package angel food cake mix
- 1 (6 ounces) package strawberry flavoured Jell-O®
- 1 (16 ounces) package of frozen strawberries
- 1 (12 ounces) container of frozen whipped topping, thawed
- 2 cups boiling water
- 1 cup water

Directions:
- ➢ In a large mixing basin, combine flavoured gelatin and boiling water, stirring until dissolved. Next, incorporate cold water and frozen strawberries. Chill until somewhat thickened, similar to egg whites. If you add a lot of frozen strawberries, it could get to this level while stirring.
- ➢ Cut the cake into cubes or rip it into bite-size portions, then trim the dark brown edges. Fold in the frozen whipped topping and cake gently into the strawberry mixture. Chill until completely set. Top with any remaining toppings and strawberries.

Dessert Bars

Preparation Time: 10 minutes

Cooking Time: 15 minutes
Servings: 1

Ingredients:
- 2 cups butter, softened
- 2 cups white sugar
- Four egg yolks
- 4 cups all-purpose flour
- 1 ½ cups raspberry jam

Directions:
- ➢ Preheat the oven carefully to 350°F (175 degrees C). Grease a 9x13 baking dish.
- ➢ Cream the butter and sugar together in a medium mixing bowl until light and creamy. Incorporate the egg yolks. Mix in the flour gradually to produce a dough. Press half of the dough into the bottom of the prepared pan using lightly greased hands. Spread raspberry jam equally over the top. To cover the top, flatten pieces of the remaining dough and arrange them on top of the raspberry layer.
- ➢ Bake for 30 minutes, or until gently brown, in a preheated oven. Allow cooling somewhat before slicing into bars.

Dessert Pizza

Preparation Time: 10 minutes
Cooking Time: 15 minutes
Servings: 1

Ingredients:
- 1 (18 ounces) package of refrigerated sugar cookie dough
- 1 (8 ounces) container of frozen whipped topping, thawed
- ½ cup sliced banana
- ½ cup sliced fresh strawberries
- ½ cup crushed pineapple, drained
- ½ cup seedless grapes halved

Directions:
- ➢ Preheat the oven carefully to 350°F (175 degrees C).
- ➢ Fill a 12-inch pizza pan halfway with cookie batter—Bake for 15 to 20 minutes, or until golden brown, in a preheated oven. Allow cooling in the pan on a wire rack.
- ➢ Spread whipped topping on top of the chilled crust. Decoratively arrange the fruit. Place in the refrigerator until ready to serve.

Postre de Limon (Mexican Lime Dessert)

Preparation Time: 10 minutes
Cooking Time: 15 minutes
Servings: 1

Ingredients:
- 1 (14 ounces) can sweeten condensed milk
- 1 (14 ounces) can evaporate milk
- Two limes, zested and juiced
- 1 (7 ounces) package of Mexican Maria cookies (galletas Maria)

Directions:
- ➢ Combine condensed milk, evaporated milk, and lime juice; beat with an electric mixer until thoroughly combined.
- ➢ In the bottom of a small baking dish, stack Maria's cookies. Cover with another layer of the milk mixture. Layer the cookies and milk mixture again, finishing with the milk mixture. Wrap the baking dish in plastic wrap. Refrigerate for 5 hours overnight or until firm.
- ➢ Cut the dough into squares. Garnish with lime zest if desired.

Pumpkin Cream Cheese Dessert

Preparation Time: 10 minutes
Cooking Time: 15 minutes
Servings: 1

Ingredients:
- ½ cup butter
- ⅓ cup white sugar

- 24 graham crackers, crushed
- Two eggs
- ¾ cup white sugar
- 1 (8 ounces) package of cream cheese, softened
- One envelope (1 tablespoon) of unflavored gelatin
- ¼ cup water
- 1 (15 ounces) can of pumpkin
- Three eggs, separated
- ½ cup milk
- ½ cup white sugar
- ½ teaspoon salt
- Two teaspoons of ground cinnamon
- ½ pint whipped cream

Directions:
- ➢ Preheat the oven carefully to 350°F (175 degrees C). Grease a 9x13-inch baking dish lightly.
- ➢ Melt butter in a medium saucepan over medium heat. Mix in the sugar well. Mix in the graham cracker crumbs. Fill a baking dish halfway with the mixture.
- ➢ Combine the eggs, sugar, and cream cheese in a medium mixing basin. Pour the mixture on top of the crust.
- ➢ Cook for 20 minutes in a preheated oven. Remove from the heat and set aside to cool.
- ➢ Dissolve the gelatin with water in a small dish.
- ➢ Combine the pumpkin, eggs, milk, sugar, salt, and cinnamon in a medium saucepan. Set aside the egg whites. Cook until thick, approximately 4 minutes, stirring regularly. Take the pan off the heat and stir in the gelatin. Allow around 20 minutes for the mixture to cool.
- ➢ In a small mixing bowl, whip the three egg whites until firm. Fold the egg whites into the cooled pumpkin mixture gently. Over the cream cheese mixture, pour the pumpkin mixture. Finish with whipped cream. Refrigerate for 2 hours, covered.

Capirotada (Mexican Dessert)

Preparation Time: 10 minutes
Cooking Time: 15 minutes
Servings: 1

Ingredients:
- 3 cups water
- 16 ounces piloncillo (Mexican brown sugar cone), chopped
- Three cinnamon sticks
- Two tablespoons of raw sugar
- Two tablespoons of vanilla extract
- ¼ teaspoon ground cloves
- ¼ cup butter
- 1 (18 ounces) loaf of French bread, sliced
- 1 ½ cup shredded Monterey Jack cheese
- 1 ½ cup chopped walnuts
- ½ cup raisins
- ½ cup chopped dried apricots

Directions:
- ➢ Preheat the oven carefully to 350° F. (175 degrees C).
- ➢ Combine water, piloncillo, cinnamon sticks, sugar, vanilla essence, and cloves in a saucepan. Bring the water to a boil—Cook for 10 minutes, or until slightly thickened and reduced to a syrup. Take out the cinnamon sticks.
- ➢ Butter each slice of bread lightly. Put the slices in a big, flat baking dish.
- ➢ 10 to 15 minutes in a preheated oven until toasted. Allow the butter to dry.
- ➢ Grease a 9x13-inch cake pan with cooking spray and add 1/2 of the toasted bread. Sprinkle the toast with 1/2 of the Monterey Jack cheese, walnuts, raisins, and apricots. Drizzle 1/2 of the syrup over the bread to properly cover it. Add the remaining bread, cheese, walnuts, raisins, apricots, and syrup to the top. Wrap with aluminium foil.

- ➢ Bake for 20 minutes in a preheated oven. Remove the foil and bake for another 15 minutes, or until gently browned and cooked through. Serve hot.

Cherry Pretzel Dessert

Preparation Time: 10 minutes
Cooking Time: 15 minutes
Servings: 1

Ingredients:
- 2 cups crushed pretzels
- ½ cup butter, melted
- Three tablespoons of white sugar
- 1 (8 ounces) package of cream cheese, softened
- 1 cup confectioners' sugar
- 1 (12 ounces) container of frozen whipped topping (such as Cool Whip®), thawed
- 1 (21 ounces) can of cherry pie filling

Directions:
- ➢ Preheat the oven carefully to 350°F (175 degrees C).
- ➢ In a mixing basin, combine pretzels, melted butter, and sugar; press into the bottom of a 13x9-inch baking dish.
- ➢ Bake the crust in a preheated oven for about 10 minutes or until gently browned. Allow cooling completely before removing.
- ➢ In a mixing basin, combine cream cheese and confectioners' sugar. Combine the whipped topping and cream cheese mixture in a mixing bowl until smooth; pour over the chilled pretzel shell. Cover the cream cheese layer with the cherry pie filling.

Tiramisu Dessert

Preparation Time: 10 minutes
Cooking Time: 15 minutes
Servings: 1

Ingredients:
- 1 cup brewed espresso
- 1 cup white sugar, divided
- ¼ cup coffee liqueur
- 1 (16 ounces) container of mascarpone cheese
- Four extra-large egg yolks
- Two tablespoons of sweet Marsala wine
- One tablespoon of coffee liqueur
- 1 cup heavy cream
- 1 (14 ounces) package of ladyfingers
- ¼ cup unsweetened cocoa powder

Directions:
- ➢ In a heavy saucepan over medium-high heat, combine espresso, 1/2 cup sugar, and 1/4 cup coffee liqueur. Simmer for 3 to 4 minutes, constantly whisking, until the sugar melts. Remove from heat and set aside to cool.
- ➢ In the bowl of a stand mixer fitted with the whisk attachment, combine the remaining 1/2 cup sugar, mascarpone cheese, egg yolks, Marsala, and the remaining one tablespoon coffee liqueur; beat on medium speed for 7 minutes, or until light and airy. Clean the mixer bowl and whisk attachment, and transfer to another basin.
- ➢ In a mixing basin, whisk heavy cream until firm peaks form. Fold the cream into the mascarpone-Marsala mixture gently.
- ➢ Take 40 ladyfingers from the packet and save the rest for later use. Dip ladyfingers one at a time into the cooled espresso syrup and place it on an 8x12-inch pan in a single layer. Half of the cream mixture should be poured on top.

Next, dip more ladyfingers and stack them perpendicularly. Top with the remaining cream mixture.
- ➢ Tiramisu should be dusted with cocoa powder. Refrigerate for at least two hours before serving.

Mombasa Pumpkin Dessert

Preparation Time: 10 minutes
Cooking Time: 15 minutes
Servings: 1

Ingredients:
- medium sugar pumpkin, seeded and cubed
- 2 cups white sugar
- 1 cup coconut milk
- One teaspoon of ground cardamom

Directions:
- ➢ For 5 to 10 minutes, steam the pumpkin chunks. Remove meat from skins.
- ➢ Combine the pumpkin flesh and sugar in a medium pot. Cook over medium-low heat until the sugar melts into the pumpkin. Mix in the coconut and cardamom. Stir often. Cook until the mixture has thickened to the consistency of thick pudding.

Easy Nesquik Butterfinger Dessert

Preparation Time: 10 minutes
Cooking Time: 15 minutes
Servings: 1

Ingredients:
- 1 ½ cup whipping cream
- ½ cup NESTLE® NESQUIK™ Chocolate Flavor Syrup
- 36 pieces Butterfinger® Bites Candy, finely chopped, divided
- 30 graham cracker squares

Directions:
- ➢ In a large mixing basin, whip the cream until soft peaks form. Beat in 1/4 cup Nesquik at a time until stiff peaks form. 1 cup Butterfinger bits, stirred in
- ➢ One heaping spoonful of whipped cream mixture equally spread over each of 6 graham cracker pieces; stack. Place the graham crackers vertically on a large plate or baking sheet. The remaining graham crackers and whipped cream mixture are repeated to make five stacks. Form a loaf by pressing stacks together.
- ➢ Cover the top and edges of the graham cracker loaf with the remaining whipped cream mixture. Finish with the remaining Butterfinger pieces.
- ➢ Refrigerate for at least two hours, preferably overnight. To serve, cut the bread diagonally into 1-inch pieces. Place a piece on each dish and drizzle with the remaining Nesquik.

Avocado Dessert

Preparation Time: 10 minutes
Cooking Time: 15 minutes
Servings: 1

Ingredients:
- One avocado, peeled and pitted
- ½ cup milk
- ¼ cup white sugar
- ½ teaspoon vanilla extract

Directions:
- ➢ Use an electric mixer or a food processor to mash the avocado. Mix in the milk, sugar, and vanilla extract until smooth. Allow for a 20-minute chill before serving.

Meal Plan

WEEK-1

Breakfast

AVOCADO SMOOTHIE	31
CHOCOLATE PEANUT BUTTER BANANA SMOOTHIES	32
ISLAND SMOOTHIE	32
ACAI BERRY SMOOTHIE	32
STRAWBERRY FIELDS SMOOTHIE	32
YAM SMOOTHIE	32
BLUE GRAPEFRUIT SMOOTHIE	32

Lunch

ALYSIA'S BASIC MEAT LASAGNA	61
MEAT PIE	61
GOOD OLD MEAT PIE	61
HALLOWEEN MEAT HEAD	61
ARGENTINE MEAT EMPANADAS	62
EASTER MEAT PIE	62
NATCHITOCHES MEAT PIES	62

Dinner

DILLY CHICKEN	56
CHEESY CHICKEN SPAGHETTI	57
EASY CHICKEN MARSALA	57
HAPPY ROAST CHICKEN	57
CHEESY CHICKEN SPAGHETTI	57
EASY CHICKEN MARSALA	58
TACO MEAT	60

WEEK-2

Breakfast

QUICK PINA COLADA SMOOTHIE	32
ALMOND BUTTER SMOOTHIE	32
GRAPEFRUIT SMOOTHIE	33
SUMMERTIME FRUIT SMOOTHIE	33
SOUR SMOOTHIE	33
CARROT-BANANA SMOOTHIE	33
STRAWBERRY BANANA BREEZE SMOOTHIE	33

Lunch

INDIAN BARBEQUE CHICKEN	54
YELLOW CHICKEN	54
CHICKEN ROTINI SOUP	54
GRILLED CHICKEN AND HERBS	54
CHICKEN SOUP	54

ITALIAN CHICKEN CACCIATORE	55
FRIED CHICKEN	55

Dinner

CHICKEN YAKISOBA	55
JUICY CHICKEN	55
CREAMY CHICKEN AND NOODLES	55
SHOYU CHICKEN	56
CHINESE GARLIC CHICKEN	56
BUFFALO CHICKEN SAUCE	56
CURRIED CHICKEN	56

WEEK-3

Breakfast

VIRGIN MARY SMOOTHIES	31
SECRET INGREDIENT SMOOTHIE	31
CRUNCHY PINEAPPLE SMOOTHIE	31
BLUEBERRY AND SPICE SMOOTHIE	31
VANILLA PUMPKIN PIE SMOOTHIE	31
AVOCADO SMOOTHIE	31
ULTIMATE FRUIT SMOOTHIE	31

Lunch

GROUND TURKEY SOUP WITH BEANS	41

CREAM OF ASPARAGUS SOUP I	42
BEST BUTTERNUT SQUASH SOUP EVER	42
QUICK CREAMY ZUCCHINI SOUP	42
THE WORLD'S BEST TORTILLA SOUP	42
CHILLED ZUCCHINI SOUP	43
KALE LASAGNA WITH MEAT SAUCE	59

Dinner

BLUE CHEESE, SPINACH MEAT LOAF MUFFINS	59
SYRIAN RICE WITH MEAT	59
DEER MEAT	59
SICILIAN MEAT ROLL	59
MONKEY MEAT	60
LAYERED TACO DIP WITH MEAT	60
POLISH MEAT AND POTATOES	60

WEEK-4

Breakfast

SILKY STRAWBERRY SMOOTHIE	33
FRUIT SMOOTHIE II	33
SILKY STRAWBERRY SMOOTHIE	33
FRUIT SMOOTHIE II	33
SILKY STRAWBERRY SMOOTHIE	34
FRUIT SMOOTHIE II	34

RASPBERRY AND APRICOT SMOOTHIE	34

Lunch

BAKED CORN TORTILLA STRIPS FOR MEXICAN SOUPS	39
FABULOUS ROASTED CAULIFLOWER SOUP	39
SLOW COOKER FRESH VEGETABLE-BEEF-BARLEY SOUP	39
POTATO SOUP	39
FENNEL SOUP	39
LEEK AND FENNEL SOUP	39
OXTAIL SOUP I	40

Dinner

COLD CUCUMBER SOUP	40
CREAM OF FRESH TOMATO SOUP	40
BASIC CHICKEN STOCK	40
HOMEMADE VEGETABLE BEEF SOUP	41
STEAK SOUP	41
CHICKEN AND GNOCCHI SOUP	41
CHICKEN VEGETABLE BARLEY SOUP	41